The Silent Passage

MENOPAUSE

The Silent Passage

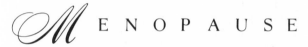ENOPAUSE

Gail Sheehy

RANDOM HOUSE　NEW YORK

Library of Congress Cataloging-in-Publication Data
Sheehy, Gail.
The silent passage : menopause / by Gail Sheehy.
            p.   cm.
Includes index.
ISBN 0-679-41388-X
1. Menopause—Psychological aspects.   2. Menopause—
Social aspects.   I. Title.
RG186.S665   1992
618.1'75052—dc20   91-51064

Manufactured in the United States of America
8 9

The text of this book is set in Linotype Walbaum
Book design by Lilly Langotsky

Author's Note

This book has two wellsprings. The first was my own ignorance. About pregnancy we are taught everything one could want to know. I remember readily finding books on natural childbirth in the library and teaching myself the breathing exercises, so that by the time I went into labor I felt fully prepared. By contrast, I went into menopause knowing nothing—not even that I was in it. Like so many women who have always enjoyed good health and who prided myself, upon reaching my mid-forties, on having achieved a fair degree of control over my life, I was sure I would just "sail right through it." Instead, I veered off course, lost some of the wind in my sails, and almost capsized.

But in trying to learn or talk about menopause, I found myself up against a powerful and mysterious taboo. My friends were adrift in the same fog of inexcusable ignorance. We couldn't help one another because none of us knew enough. Putting on my investigative journalist's hat, I explored the state of knowledge on menopause in this country, Canada, and Europe and was appalled to find how backward we are in basic research on a condition that is hardly new. After some thought, I decided to break the taboo and go public with my own, not uncommon experience and found other well-known women willing to do the same. *Vanity Fair* published my article in October 1991.

The immediate and electrifying response to that article was a further impetus to write this book. The fears and frustrations expressed had clearly struck a nerve much deeper than I had imagined, and more than a hundred letters with detailed comments served as an alert that there was more to be done. One letter gave testimony to the stigma we are passing on to our daughters by succumbing to the silence.

> I'm only 20 years old and never really understood what menopause was. I understood it was the time in a woman's life when she went batty for a couple of years and slowly but surely lost it upstairs. I now have a better understanding of what it is, as well as a great respect and sympathy for every woman that goes through it.
> —Elise Starr, Vancouver, B.C., Canada

For this book I made a commitment to listen to women, to record their experiences with the Change of Life, hoping their stories will act as the catalyst for honest conversations about menopause between mothers and daughters, wives and husbands, women and their doctors. Of the scanty research on menopause, almost none has reached beyond well-educated white women who live near academic centers or who have the means to consult doctors about health maintenance at this time of life. What about all the rest—don't they have menopause, too?

To seek out women from all social levels and races and regions of the United States I conducted intimate group interviews, as well as collected individual life histories, in places as dissimilar as Eugene, Oregon; Rochester, New York; Louisville, Kentucky; downtown Los Angeles and Beverly Hills in California; Queens and Manhattan in New York. Participants included privileged women and low-income government workers, women of color and polite white suburbanites, mid-forties women antic- ipating the Change and women in their sixties who could look back on it with some perspective. In all, I interviewed over one hundred women in various stages of menopause. The emphasis in this book is on their vivid and varied experiences of this silent passage.

More detailed medical information was also necessary to raise awareness among women as health consumers. In my research I freely crossed disciplines, reaching be- yond the obvious medical practitioners—gynecologists, breast surgeons, and internists—to endocrinologists, who study the hard science of hormones, and epidemiologists, who measure all the factors contributing to a condition like menopause in large populations. Additional light was shed on this complex life transition by interviews with research physiologists, neuroscientists, psycholo- gists, psychiatrists, and gerontologists; and practical ap- proaches to coping with it were suggested by nutritionists and Chinese medicine doctors. For a larger historical and evolutionary perspective I consulted scholars in sociology and anthropology, historians, and primate researchers. I interviewed a total of seventy-five experts.

I was not altogether alone in my explorations. Patricia Allen, an obstetrician-gynecologist in private practice in Manhattan and on the staff at New York Hospital, took an interest in my efforts—both as my personal doctor and as a professional committed to expanding health education for women. Dr. Allen introduced me to top specialists in related fields, and I discussed with her the findings of scientists that challenged status quo gynecological practice. Finally she took to the trenches with me to listen in on some of the group interviews in other parts of the country. It was a journey of discovery that helped me, as cultural translator, to shed stereotypes and orthodoxies. I am indebted to Dr. Allen for offering meticulous professional companionship in the final production of this book.

My thanks also go to Dr. William J. Ledger, professor and chairman of Obstetrics and Gynecology at the New York Hospital–Cornell Medical Center, and to Dr. Robert Lindsay, a leading research endocrinologist in the field of menopause medicine and practitioner at the Helen Hayes Bone Center, both of whom read the manuscript and added suggestions and refinements. It has been my privilege to work with one of the country's most distinguished editors, Robert Loomis, and my good fortune to have the assistance of Leora Tanenbaum.

The women who gallantly contributed their personal stories to this book are also my partners. Some of their names and backgrounds had to be altered, but others offered their real names. To each I offer thanks for striking one more small blow for normalization of a proud stage of life.

Contents

─────

The Silent Passage

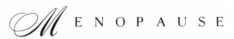

ENOPAUSE

"The Need to Know
and the
Fear of Knowing"

A group of recognizably high-powered media women on the shady side of forty were spaced around the table between their husbands and lovers at a Washington dinner party when a single sentence shattered their well-groomed calm. It came out of the mouth of the stunning network newswoman who ordinarily speaks in ninety-second bursts of inside-the-Beltway shorthand.

"Okay, there are only two subjects worth talking about—menopause and face-lifts." It was as though a nine-hundred-pound gorilla had just jumped up on the table.

We think of ourselves as so liberated today that we can talk about anything. People will tell strangers about their abortions or alcoholism, even declare on national television that they are HIV positive with the AIDS virus, yet women still shrink from mentioning, even to their good women friends, the fear they might be menopausal. And just let a man suggest to his sleepless, perspiry, weepy wife that her uncharacteristic moods and symptoms might have something to do with menopause; he's bound to get a blanket denial: "What are you talking about! I'm too young!"

Menopause may be the last taboo. The first friend to whom I mentioned the subject is a sultry-looking woman of fifty (pre–baby boom). She has always prided herself on her appearance and gained much of her status from creatively supporting her husband, a successful author who looks somewhat younger than she. I asked if she had ever talked with anyone about menopause.

"No. And I don't want to."

"Women don't bring up the subject around you?"

"One friend did," she said sourly. "I haven't seen her since."

Another friend, a public television producer whose natural temperament is appallingly calm, recalled with rueful laughter her first sign of the Change of Life. She was seated between two titans of industry at a high-protocol Park Avenue dinner party, the kind where the place cards look like tracings from the *Book of Kells*, and she was feeling particularly confident and pretty in her new black designer suit with its flattering white satin collar when out of the blue a droplet of something hit her collar. Then another drop. What the—was the help dribbling wine? Could there be a leaky ceiling under all that gorgeous boiserie? Suddenly she noticed her husband's gaze turn to alarm from across the table: What horrible thing was happening to her? She put a hand to her face. Her forehead was wet as a swamp.

Oh, no, said her eyes, *not me!* as the moisture began

running in rivulets down her face and slipping off her chin—*plop*—onto her pearly satin collar. *Should I pick up the white linen napkin and wipe my forehead?* She reached for the five-hundred-threads-per-inch napery, hesitated—*no, all the makeup will come off on the damn napkin*—when a few more plops fell into her décolletage. Frantic, she began dabbing at her face. Trying to pretend it wasn't happening, she turned to her dinner partner and began smiling and mopping, chatting and fanning, laughing at his jokes and dabbing, trying to keep up her end of the conversation while she wanted nothing more in this world than to disappear into the kitchen and tear off her clothes and open the freezer door—never mind that it was February—and just *stand there.*

That was a year ago. She and her husband have had the Thermostat Wars usual in menopausal households— "It's freezing in here!" "No, it's boiling." "Did you turn the thermostat below fifty again?" "Oh, why don't you just get some flannel pajamas!" But the producer is one of the lucky ones: She has had no other indicators beyond hot flashes that she is passing into another stage of life.

It happens to every woman. Pregnancy we can choose to go through or not. With menopause there is no choice. It happens to teachers and discount store clerks and dental hygienists, who nonetheless have to function in public, on their feet, every day. It happens to Navy pilots and gray-haired graduate students and former Olympic athletes, who are accustomed to demanding the highest physical and mental performance from themselves. It happens to women of color, to women in the home, to women of glamour like Jackie O. Indeed, the most powerful woman in the world throughout the decade of the

Eighties was a menopausal woman. Margaret Thatcher broke the glass ceiling in British politics, becoming leader of the Conservative party just as she was about to hit fifty. She went through menopause while making the leap to world leader. It happens even in Hollywood. Raquel and Farrah and Ann-Margret, too, must deal with menopause. These women are hardly over the hill. In fact, they are hitting a new stride.

But they never mention the big M.

Ironically, the people who are the most evasive and unsympathetic about menopause tend to be those closest to it—women in their mid to late forties—who can be "menophobic." Their own resistance to identifying with the stage of life beyond reproductivity is sometimes expressed in an uncharacteristic intolerance of their own friends.

A thirty-nine-year-old Chicago woman moved to a new city the year her premature menopause came on. Although she made new friends quickly, they began to shun her as soon as she mentioned physical signs associated with the Change of Life. The ostracized woman struggled through five years with a large fibroid cyst, digestive problems, eating only mashed potatoes, and losing twenty pounds, before her friends and doctors acknowledged the source of her difficulties.

"I clearly remember not being sympathetic," recalled one of her best friends with considerable regret. Other of the woman's friends recalled their impatience. "We'd talk about her among ourselves: 'She's complaining about hot flashes and stomach problems again this week. Why doesn't she just get over it?' We never really said, 'She's suffering.' We certainly never mentioned the possibility of menopause. And here we are, *women*."

"Women can be the worst," acknowledged her best friend. The formerly shunned woman now realizes, "People wouldn't relate my problems to menopause because that would automatically classify them as old."

Shame, fear, misinformation—and, most of all, the stigma of aging in a youth-obsessed society—are the vague demons that have kept us silent about a passage that could not be more universal among females. The most common fears are: *I'll lose my looks, I'll lose my sex appeal, I'll get depressed, fade into the woodwork, I'll become invisible.* We don't have to lose any of these things. Yet all of the obvious sources of information and comfort—mothers, doctors, the media, academics—have shied away from the subject. It's as though there has been a conspiracy of silence. No one wants us to find out how much power we have. All that is about to change.

Right now the number of American women in peri-menopause (the term used to designate the transition phase between regular periods and no periods at all), in menopause, or past menopause totals *forty-three million.* And the next decade will see an explosion in the menopausal population in the United States: The number of women between the ages of forty-five and fifty-four will increase by half, from thirteen million to nineteen million. The sheer numbers may at last confer normalcy on this predictable passage.

I know what you're thinking. *Thank God this is a book that I don't have to read.* Because you're not fifty yet, or even close. That's the first misconception.

"Y O U ' R E   N O T

O L D   E N O U G H"

Murphy Brown may be having a baby in her forties, but Candice Bergen, who plays her on TV, is beginning to think about the Change of Life. The ravishing forty-six-year-old, having married late and blossomed as both a mother and a comedienne in her fifth decade, feels the shock of time compression. It came out in an interview with Jane Pauley on *Real Life*: "I saw this article on menopause in a magazine and I went, well, I don't need to look at *that*." And she wrinkled her Scandinavian ski-jump nose. "And then I thought, 'Oh, my *God*! Is this what's coming? Is this what's next? We have to deal with menopause? At my age? But I'm a *kid*.' "

Menopause is arbitrarily defined as "the final cessation of menstruation," as if it were a single point in time when the switch is turned off on those fabulous egg-ripening machines, the ovaries. In fact, it's a much more gradual, stop-start series of pauses in ovarian function that are part of that mysterious process called aging. (A more comprehensive term is the climacteric, for which there is a male counterpart.) We are born with all the eggs we'll ever have, about seven hundred thousand. Each month after puberty, one ovary offers up a selection of from twenty to one thousand mature eggs, though usually only one is released into the fallopian tube to meet any sperm in the vicinity. As we get close to the bottom of the egg basket, ovulation doesn't always take place. The quality of egg follicles that month may be substandard, or there

may not be sufficient estrogen manufactured by the ovaries. When the supply of viable eggs is gone, menstruation
stops completely and the fertile period of a woman's life
ends.

The median age at which women in Western countries
stop ovulating altogether is 50.8. But today there are no
clear age cues to when the long transition begins or when
it ends. "For a long time we've thought of menopause as
a very sudden event—it really isn't," says Dr. Trudy Bush,
epidemiologist and associate professor of obstetrics and
gynecology at Johns Hopkins Medical School. "The ovaries start producing less estrogen probably in the mid-
thirties. There's a gradual loss of estrogen production and
other hormones until the ovaries finally stop putting out
very much estrogen at all. It's not uncommon to see symptoms in the early forties as a sign of gradual estrogen
withdrawal."

Increasingly, say veteran practitioners, the American
women turning up in menopause clinics are younger by
four or five years than in the recent past. Researchers
now admit they have underestimated the number of
younger women who experience all the symptoms of
menopause even though they still have periods. "We
know now there are women who start experiencing
changes in their menstrual cycle in their late thirties,"
says Phyllis Kernoff Mansfield, a veteran researcher of
female cycles at Penn State.

My own younger sister started missing periods when
she was forty-three—five years earlier than it began with
me. One month her "little friend" would come, then not
again for another two or three months, whereupon it
would reappear, only to disappear again. After half a year

of this, feeling poorly, she called her gynecologist and popped the obvious question: "Is this the beginning of menopause?"

"No," he stated categorically. "You're not old enough."

It's tempting to take this sop so commonly put out by physicians and to go away feeling smug and secure in one's continuing fecundity. Isn't it reassuring to know that you're still young? Well, not *young* exactly, but still, in some respect at least, *underage*.

"I started very early, at forty," I was told by another woman I'll call Barbara, a delightfully wise Oregonian with a thriving psychotherapy practice. "It was no fun. I was blown away by the hot flashes. I felt enormous restlessness, and cranky, cranky, cranky!" Her doctor, too, said she wasn't old enough to take estrogen. Or, as she heard it, she hadn't suffered enough.

A roaring extrovert, Barbara stood up to her full five feet nine inches and stared down her doctor. "Either you give me estrogen, or the next time I have a hot flash I'm going to rip my clothes off and shout your name!"

The man dispensed the pills and preserved his anonymity, but once on hormones, Barbara blew up. "I gained five pounds a year for six years until I finally said the hell with it. I quit taking the estrogen, and I have all the lines in my face to show for it." Now in her early fifties, she does look parched and abruptly elderly. "You age faster after menopause," she concludes, though it would be more accurate to say one ages faster after any *abrupt* withdrawal from hormones.

On the opposite end, women may never be quite sure when, or if, they have finished with menopause. This is particularly true for women who go right onto hormone therapy at the first signs of the Change and continue having periods as if they were still reproductive. There is no noticeable evidence of when they stop ovulating, no clear metaphysical marker that they are moving beyond fertility into another stage of life.

Margaret Mead originated the memorable phrase *post-menopausal zest.* Yet Mary Catherine Bateson, the daughter of the pioneering anthropologist, is still puzzled about when her own mother actually became menopausal. When Dr. Mead reached the age of forty-eight and probably experienced the first hot flashes, she persuaded her doctor to try giving her shots of estrogen, the primary female hormone, telling him it was for a circulatory problem. "And it worked," she noted in a brief medical history made available to me by her daughter, an anthropological researcher and author in her own right. At age fifty-three Dr. Mead noted "longer space between periods and lighter flow." But she continued to have hormone-induced periods for another eight years, whereupon she asserted that she had held off menopause until her sixties.

To add to the age blurring, vanguard baby boomers are giving birth to yet another phenomenon unique to their generation: *menopause moms.* A woman I'll call Sondra had been involved in SDS at Columbia—"a classic sixties person," as she described herself. She spent the next fifteen years as a politically obsessed radical in "movement work," followed by a very respectable marriage and a cascade of miscarriages. Sondra was forty-two by the time she finally produced her first baby. That was two years ago.

"Thank God I finished breast feeding just in time for menopause," she deadpanned. She swears she felt hot flashes while she was breast feeding (a normal occurrence).

Over the next few years the boardrooms of America are going to light up with hot flashes. The point women among the baby boomers, those now in their mid-forties who are the first among their generation to approach the passage into menopause, are probably operating at 110 percent. They may be in command positions in their professional lives, or starting over to get a graduate degree, while also feeling a new sense of social obligation. Those who have remained childless and had conflicted feelings about it can turn their care-giving instincts outward. The married ones have a new chance for romance with a neglected husband, if the nest is now empty; the divorced or widowed ones may choose to savor their independence or delight in a new love or a new sexual orientation. But at the same time, many women over forty-five are likely to be sandwiched between an abruptly dependent parent or in-law who is entering the twilight of ill health and the continued dependence of children who today remain adolescent until the end of their twenties—and even move back in! This is no time suddenly to find one can't sleep, or can't shake the blues, or lacks the old zip.

Moreover, acute or prolonged stress can affect a woman's cycle at any point in her life. Top literary agent Lynn Nesbit has an exceptionally demanding career, which helped precipitate a very sudden change in her cycle. Somewhat nonplussed, she went to her gynecologist, a venerated Park Avenue practitioner who had seen her through the birth of her two children ("I see him as my savior"). He told her she should have a D&C, after which her cycle disappeared for four months. When she was next examined, the doctor announced that her hormone level had fallen drastically. She had just turned fifty. The doctor wanted to put her on Premarin and Provera, the usual combined-hormone therapy.

Being an exceptionally healthy, dynamic woman and disciplined about diet and exercise, Nesbit was nervous about this advice; after all, there was the well-publicized risk of breast cancer. "I thought, oh, God, I don't know if I want to just pop hormones." Then she thought about her youthful-looking seventy-five-year-old mother, who has never gone a day for three decades without her Premarin. And her doctor added to all the conventional reasons a couple that were new and thought-provoking: "It keeps your memory, and you don't wrinkle as badly."

That sold her. "I look at three of my friends who *don't* take hormones and their skin looks like leather." So, never having experienced a hot flash or any change in energy level, the superagent has temporarily detoured around this profound passage or at least the immediate physical experience of it. Like many women who choose hormone therapy and are lucky enough to adjust to it easily, Nesbit can say, "No, I don't consider myself a menopausal woman. I never even think about it."

More than one third of the women in the United States have hysterectomies—thirty-seven women out of one hundred—an astounding figure. (North America leads the world in numbers of hysterectomies, with twice as many as in Great Britain.) The majority of these women have hysterectomies between the ages of twenty-five and forty-four. Hysterectomy alone, which means removal of the uterus and cervix, rarely produces menopause. However, removal of the ovaries, called oophorectomy, brings on menopause immediately, no matter how young a woman is.

This is all part of a fundamental change in the way we view the adult life cycle of women. *The biological transition of menopause is no longer an age-tied marker event.*

But no matter when the first awareness dawns on a woman that menopause might be imminent for *her*, it comes as a shock. Virtually nothing prepares most women for this mysterious and momentous transition. Indeed, some of us unconsciously tell ourselves, "It's not going to happen to me."

WHEN YOU LEAST EXPECT IT

No more incongruous time or place could be imagined, the night I was hit by the first bombshell of the battle with menopause. It was a Sunday evening. Snug inside a remarriage not yet a year old, I was sitting utterly still, reading, in a velvet-covered armchair. A pillow's throw away my husband was doing the same, while jazz lapped at our ears and snow curtained the window. Every so often we looked up and congratulated ourselves on staying home in this cocoon of comfort and safeness and love we had created.

Then the little grenade went off in my brain. A flash, a shock, a sudden surge of electrical current that whizzed through my head and left me feeling shaken, nervous, off-balance.

"What was that?" I must have mumbled.

"What?"

"Nothing."

But some powerful switch had been thrown. I tried to go back to reading. It was difficult to concentrate. When I looked down at the pages I had just finished, I realized the imprint of their content on my brain had washed out. I felt hot, then clammy. I tried lying down, but sleep could not soak up the agitation. My heart was racing, but from what? Complete repose? I felt, for perhaps the first time in my life since the age of thirteen, profoundly ill at ease inside my body.

In the months that followed, I sometimes felt *outside* my body. I was aware of spates of "static" in my brain and came to recognize the aura that preceded the first migraine-like headaches I'd ever had. Usually optimistic, I began having little bouts of blues. Then little crashes of fatigue. Having always counted on abundant energy, it was profoundly upsetting to find myself sometimes crawling home from a day of writing and falling into bed for a "nap," from which I had to drag myself up just to have dinner.

I was only forty-eight. And still menstruating. So this couldn't be "Change of Life," could it?

Besides, all these strange physical sensations were only background noise in what was otherwise a thrilling, adrenaline-pumping, mind-stretching period of creative redirection, in both my career and my new family life. I was traveling all over the country and the world and coming home to a husband and new adopted child, both of whom I adored. So I took Scarlett's "fiddledeedee" approach; I'd think about it tomorrow.

But tomorrow I began to notice something strange. For the first time since my early teens, when the sexual pilot light went on and I was warned not to want sex too much, I began to worry about not wanting it enough. Again, I had the sensation of standing outside my body and scolding it: "What's the matter with you—why don't you *act* the way I feel anymore?"

I went to see my conservative, male gynecologist, known as a superb clinician but short on communication skills. He measured my hormone levels. I was very low on estrogen. I vaguely remembered my family doctor having mentioned in passing, when he'd rattled off the results of my annual physical in recent years, that my estrogen levels were getting lower and lower.

"Could I be a candidate for hormone replacement therapy?" I asked.

"Not yet." My gynecologist went strictly by the book. "You're not in menopause, because you're still menstruating. You have to be menstruation-free for a year before I can give you estrogen replacement."

"But this, um, effect on my sexual response"—embarrassed, I fumbled for the words—"couldn't that be because I need more estrogen, like a vitamin supplement?"

"It's nothing I can help you with. Decrease in sexual response is just a natural part of aging."

The curt clinician washed his hands of me. I left his office feeling as though I'd just been handed a one-way ticket to the Dumpster. *Does this mean I can't be me anymore?*

It was time for me to shop for another gynecologist. A recommendation sent me to see Patricia Allen, a vivacious woman in her forties and an attending physician at New York Hospital who demands excellence of herself and discipline from her patients. She made it clear from the start that she does not accept passive patients or women who smoke, only those who are willing to participate actively in their own health care. That sounded reasonable. She spent a good twenty minutes before the physical exam taking a holistic history. The irregular periods, the erratic expanding and constricting of blood vessels that caused the static, and the mood swings indicated to her that I was in perimenopause. Then she said something startling:

"I believe in treating each patient as an individual. This perimenopausal period should be a transformation, so that a woman gets to become—physically, emotionally, and spiritually—the best that she ever was." Imagine your run-of-the-mill male gynecologist harboring such a radical point of view!

Dr. Allen posited that the impact of low estrogen on me, as on many women, was emotional. Of the several hundred patients who consult her about managing their menopause, quite a few mention feeling depressed although they have no rational reason to be. She also took seriously my distress over changes in libido. She asked if there was a history of osteoporosis in my family, which brought to mind memories of my mother suffering in her seventies as she sat on her powdery bones.

All in all, Dr. Allen felt I was a good candidate for hormone therapy, but she drove a strict bargain with her patients. Estrogen by itself carries a known increase in the risk of cancer of the endometrium—the lining of the uterus, which is sloughed during menstrual periods. So she also prescribed a progestin (synthetic progesterone), reportedly a protection against that risk. Also, I would have to agree to have an endometrial biopsy several months later to detect any changes in the tissue. She also urged me to have a bone density evaluation done, as well as a mammogram. This complete diagnostic workup cost eight hundred dollars, much of which was reimbursable by health insurance. It was costly, but it turned out to be part of an investment in long-term health and productivity that has more than paid for itself—and one I would recommend for all women who can afford it.

But even this sympathetic gynecologist, like every other clinician, was unable to give definitive answers concerning the increased risk of breast cancer when one takes hormones. "We just don't know."

I filled the standardized prescription for 0.625 mg of Premarin (estrogen made from pregnant mares' urine, from which it derives its unforgettable name) and 10 mg tablets of Provera, the progestin that stimulates the sloughing of the uterine lining. This is an approximation of the two hormones that the body produces naturally in the reproductive years.

After only a month the estrogen had rekindled sexual desire, stopped the surges of static and dips of fatigue, and chased away the blues. But the Provera was another matter. It brought on unbelievable physical and emotional symptoms that I'd never experienced before. After a year of the combined hormones, my body seemed to be at war with itself for half of every month. My energy was flagging, and resistance to minor infections was falling. I felt as if I were racing my motor. So I stopped taking hormones cold turkey.

Dr. Allen agreed it was a good idea to take a break and see how the body responded. If nothing else, she said, going off hormones often serves to remind women why they started taking them in the first place.

For the first two months off hormones I felt marvelous; the bloating disappeared, as did the induced periods, and the terrible cramps and tension and sleeplessness that had begun to accompany them. I even got my waist back. Then, a crash. All the perimenopausal phenomena returned with exaggerated force. Now the static became full-fledged hot flushes and night sweats that interrupted sleep and left me limp by morning. I went back to my estrogen pills.

Within days the "blue-meanie" moods lifted. I was able to write for twelve hours straight on deadline and remain calm and reasonable under crisis. Within a few weeks all the other complaints were gone. I was staggered by the potency of the female hormone.

But the impact of the progestin was also intensified. On day fifteen, when I had to add the Provera pills to my regimen, I felt by afternoon as if I had a terrible hangover. This chemically induced state was not to be subdued by aspirin or a walk in the park. It only worsened as the day wore on, bringing with it a racing heart, irritability, waves of sadness, and difficulty concentrating. And to top it off, the hot flushes came back! Cramps introduced pain for a week at a time. By night I couldn't go to sleep without a glass of wine, and even then was awakened by a racing heartbeat and sweating. *Won't I ever be me anymore?*

It didn't require a ten-year clinical trial and double-blind study to guess what was going on. Taking synthetic progesterone with the estrogen for half of each month was like pushing down the gas pedal and putting on the brakes at the same time, and it had left my body confused and worn out.

Clinicians I later interviewed relayed common side effects reported by patients who were taking the drug: "Whenever I take Provera, I have migraines, bloating, breast tenderness, the blues. I feel awful and want to die."

No wonder fewer than 20 percent of American women in menopause are getting hormone supplements. Dr. Marc Deitch, medical director of Wyeth-Ayerst, the cash cow of the pharmaceutical giant American Home Products, which introduced Premarin fifty years ago, acknowledges that the average length of time women continue on estrogen replacement is only nine months. An estimated one third of those given prescriptions for hormones never even fill them, and two thirds of those who start out with the combination simply drop the progestin after about a year.

My little truancy was to stop taking the nasty progestin and keep on with my happy estrogen pills. However, I cut the dose in half. Dr. Allen warned me this was not conventional treatment, explaining again that in a woman with a uterus, if the supplemental estrogen is not challenged with some form of progestin, the risk of uterine cancer may increase. "We hope Provera reduces that risk, but we don't know for certain"—she frowned, as frustrated as I—"and we won't know before you've passed through this transition." We also recognized that 0.3 mg of Premarin would not offer significant support to the bones.

"Why don't you do some research on other regimens?" Dr. Allen suggested. Doctors who have done small-scale research report that progestins block some of the estrogen-receptor sites—so an internal war between the two hormones is an endocrinological reality! Progestin therefore counters some of the cardio-protective effect that is one of the most highly touted benefits of estrogen. And unlike estrogen, it offers no added protection against bone loss. A Swedish study, which showed estrogen slightly increases a woman's risk of breast cancer, fingered the addition of progestin as possibly furthering the risk—and made a big splash in *The New York Times*. The study was bitterly criticized by North American experts for drawing conclusions from too small a sample of women who were given the estrogen-progestin combination.

As for the safety of progestins, what I found out was that Provera has never been approved for treatment of menopause by the Food and Drug Administration. In fact, the FDA's Advisory Committee on Fertility and Maternal Health Drugs acknowledged that the progestins approved for hormone replacement therapy are "none." Government health officials were asked at an FDA meeting in '91: To what degree does the addition of progestin affect the possible risk of breast cancer induced by using estrogen alone? And does the addition of progestin blunt the protective effect of estrogen against heart disease and death in women? "The data are not yet adequate to permit an answer [to these questions]" was the reply. In fact, at present no data exist in North America or the United Kingdom on the impact of progestin on breast cancer risk. Notwithstanding, the FDA committee stated that this combination of hormones "may be used indefinitely by a woman with a uterus." What's more, the advisory committee was asked what proportion of the female population over age fifty would be suitable candidates for long-term consumption of estrogen alone or combined with progestin. "Virtually all." A blank check.

In 1991, $750 million of estrogen products were sold in the United States. Drug companies anticipate that these hormones will account for close to a billion-dollar market in 1992. With the baby boom bulge shifting eight hundred thousand women into the target group in '92 and projected to add over a half million women to the mid-life population each year for the rest of the decade, the menopause market is becoming big business.

"The bottom line is the right studies need to be done for the right length of time, and clearly, for economic and political reasons they're not," says Dr. Jamie Grifo, a gynecologist at New York Hospital. "Why? Who supports the majority of the research? The drug companies."

Believe it or not, no study has been completed in North America on the possible carcinogenic consequences of the combined-hormone therapy routinely prescribed for women in menopause. "Hormone replacement which includes systemic progestin . . . may be beneficial, but it is at least as likely to be harmful," concludes a review of studies by T. M. Mack at the University of Southern California. Yet over the past few years combined hormone therapy has been routinely prescribed by doctors to somewhere between four and five million American women.

Is it even conceivable that millions of men over fifty—those at the highest levels of the power structure—would be herded by physicians toward chemical dependence on powerful hormones at suspicion for causing testicular cancer? "It's the largest *un*controlled clinical trial in the history of medicine," charges public health expert Dr. Lewis Kuller. This was my introduction to the scandalous politics of menopause.

DEAL OR DENY?

My experience is not abnormal. From 10 to 15 percent of women are assumed by the few, inadequate studies to have no problems with menopause. Another 10 to 15 percent are rendered temporarily dysfunctional. The rest of us—70 percent of all women—wrestle to some degree with difficulties that come and go over a period of years as we deal with the long transition from our reproductive state. (Data going back to the nineteenth century are consistent: Almost all women experience some menopausal symptoms, but few have severe problems.)

"Menopause is not a disease," says epidemiologist Trudy Bush. "It's a life transition, but it carries with it a different internal hormonal milieu which is, in fact, detrimental to our bodies. When we don't have estrogen, our bones get brittle, our rates of heart disease go up, our vagina becomes less moist, our skin becomes dry and thin. In fact, we can reverse those processes that are related to the hormones rather than to aging per se."

The temptation, of course, is to deny the signs. Or to give up on dealing with the larger passage because we can't find quick and easy answers to resolve the physical challenge of menopause. In talking to women all over the country, I did find some significant differences in attitudes and reactions to menopause, depending on how women are valued in a particular subculture. But there was one strong common denominator: Women in midlife are afraid to know—and fiercely resist acknowledging—that menopause can affect *them*, but at the same time, in spite of themselves, they are desperately anxious to learn what it's all about. Privately they will go to extraordinary lengths to pick up information—stealing books from doctors' offices, cornering a researcher at a party and interrogating him—but heaven forbid that anyone should bring up the subject at the dinner table! Psychologist Abraham Maslow gave a name to this syndrome of ambivalence: "the need to know and the fear of knowing."

In fact, there is no one risk-free solution. Menopause is highly idiosyncratic. Remember how different we were, one from another, as we entered puberty—some of us embarrassed still to be wearing undershirts at thirteen, while our best friend was turning into a hunchback to hide the pods suddenly swelling under her sweater? Well, the Change of Life is even more individual. Peggy Sue may tell you that she hardly noticed a thing. Her periods tapered off, she had a few hot flashes, but she sailed right through—no problem. Peggy Sue may be one of the lucky 10 or 15 percent of women who find the Change of Life uneventful. She may also be plump, or obese, and since estrogen is stored in the fat cells, this is one case where fat is more advantageous than thin.

Or, she may be lying.

Whatever Peggy Sue's experience of the Change, it doesn't make *your* signs and symptoms any less true. The older we grow, the more *un*like we are, one from another. Besides the changes in our brains and sexual characteristics over the years, our endocrine systems are different, our metabolisms are different, our blood vessels and bones become more dissimilar, depending on our lifetime eating and exercise habits. So it is not surprising that there is not *one* menopause; there are hundreds of variations.

But instead of giving in to frustration over dealing with our uniqueness, we can recognize how lucky we are. In all of human history women's lives were under the coercion of their biology. Today we don't have to be forty-five years old and suddenly estrogen-deficient, miserable, and without recourse. We have choices.

The first step we can take toward mastering this stage of life is to describe the beast, give a shape and characteristics to it, and look it in the face. Incidentally, isn't it odd that an event exclusive to women begins with the word *men*? (The actual derivation of the word is from the Greek *meno*, meaning "month," and *pausis*, which is translated as "ending," though more accurately it connotes a pause in the life cycle.)

I prefer to call it the Change, because it is a change of life, one of the three great "blood mysteries" that demarcate a woman's inner life, the earlier ones being menarche and pregnancy. Despite the trial-and-error state of medical care, a woman at fifty now has a second chance. To use it, she must make an alliance with her body and negotiate with her vanity. Today's healthy, active pace-setters will become the pioneers, mapping out a whole new territory for potent living and wisdom sharing from one's fifties to one's eighties and even beyond.

Yet the reluctance to discuss both the trials and the rewards of moving through the Change of Life has ob-scured the facts, often keeping younger women in a state of menopausal dread. One naturally asks, *If menopause is such a significant passage to a whole new stage of life, why is it so neglected?*

MOTHER DOESN'T KNOW BEST

"I don't know how to be fifty," one West Coast woman told me. "I'm not going to be fifty like my mother, and there haven't really been any models."

Very rarely had any of the women I interviewed learned much about menopause from their own mothers. If they reported any mother-daughter conversation on the sub-ject at all, the mothers' answers tended to be brief and evasive: "There was nothing to it; my periods just stopped"; or, "I don't remember much about meno-pause." "When I asked my mother about menopause," said Effie Graham, a black nurse who grew up in the South, "all she said was, 'You'll find out when you get it.' She never told me about my period either."

In a longitudinal study of five hundred women graduates of a midwestern university, Professor Phyllis Mansfield found that college-educated women get their "facts" about menopause first from a friend, second from books or the media, and only third from their mothers. The last person most women consult is a doctor. One woman told a researcher she learned about menopause from Edith on an episode of *All in the Family.*

There are good reasons that the same mothers and mothers-in-law who assume possession of the revealed wisdom on child rearing are peculiarly scanty of expertise on this subject. The mothers of today's menopause-aged women came through the Depression and were an exceptionally prudish lot. It was shameful to discuss any bodily functions in their day.

And what was there to discuss about menopause? Our mothers had no information. No biomedical research had been done on the most pressing health questions of women as they age. Most of our mothers had no idea of the major killer diseases or disorders that would deprive them of a decent quality of life in their sixties, seventies, or eighties. And they certainly didn't know that their risk of being attacked by heart disease, hip fractures, and breast cancer was decidedly affected by the way they handled their Change of Life.

It is safe to assume most of our mothers never even heard the word *osteoporosis*—a silent disease caused by deterioration of the bone tissue—much less associated it with menopause. Only in the last five years or so has osteoporosis been identified as a crippler of life's quality, afflicting almost twenty-five million women. It leeches the very lining of our bones, like a colony of termites inside our foundations. Beginning their invisible destruction as soon as our supply of estrogen is depleted, these "termites" accelerate their robbing of mineral from our bones during the time around menopause.

Many women in their forties today are at the hub of several generations. Unless they're incapacitated, they feel too stretched for time and money to consult doctors or take expensive tests in order to manage their own menopause. In fact, most middle-class and low-income women don't consult any professional about how to protect their health and well-being during the Change of Life. If they adopt their mothers' attitudes without examination, they often follow blindly a path that, unbeknownst to the older women, may have been responsible for untold deficits of mental and physical well-being.

"My mother had a surgical menopause in her early forties," mentioned Gloria, a nurse from an Italian-American family, "so I really don't know much about it." Gloria herself had run into some mean symptoms starting in her forty-eighth year, which she refused to connect to menopause. "I was having terrible flashes, insomnia, I was very depressed," she described, "but I associated it with changing jobs." Although Gloria had successfully practiced pediatric nursing all her life, she found herself suddenly upset by the demands of sickly children. "I was crying all the time."

Others in the group interview asked if she had seen a doctor. "No," admitted the nurse. "I was going to coax myself out of it, be calm, take deep breaths." She explained that her mother had ingrained in her an aversion to taking any medicine, especially hormones.

Gloria had no idea if her own mother had been given estrogen after having her ovaries removed. "That's very private," she said, reflecting a common silence in ethnic families. "Even her sisters don't know." Gloria had been a nurse for almost thirty years, yet she had never stopped to wonder what it must have been like for her own mother to suffer the sudden depletion of hormones after a full hysterectomy, an experience often described as a nightmare. She had simply adhered to the voice of her inner dictator—perhaps replicating her mother's stoical misery—and denied herself permission to have any problems with the Change. In the process she almost lost her job. "I totally lost confidence in myself as a nurse," Gloria confessed. "And I didn't know that I would be able to conquer it."

In addition to the lack of informed guidance by their mothers, American women who are in the menopause years right now are handicapped by their own inhibitions. Born in the late Thirties or early Forties, they went through high school in the uptight Fifties, before the sexual revolution, before liberation, when only "bad girls" became sexually active before marriage, and a lot of others lied about it. Part of the Silent Generation, they have never been comfortable talking about sexual matters. Their silence on the subject of menopause may be an anachronism.

HISTORY AND THE
VICTORIAN HANGOVER

Another reason for the mystery surrounding menopause is that human females today are monkeying with evolution. Most higher primates do not live long enough in the wild even to have a menopause; the phenomenon has never been clearly established in apes or monkeys, according to Kim Wallen, a researcher at Emory University's Yerkes Primate Center. Most female animals just go right on breeding until they roll over and die.

The same was true of human females for many thousands of years. At the turn of the century a woman could expect to live to the age of forty-seven or -eight. She bore an average of eight children, which kept her busy giving birth or nursing right up to menopause.

Nature, then, never provided for women who would *routinely* live several decades beyond the age of fifty. Once females had made their genetic contribution, evolution was finished with them, and society followed suit. In view of this historically powerful linkage of menopause with decline and death, is it any wonder that today's women approach fifty under a shadow of archetypal fears of being transformed, all at once, into Old Woman?

The secrecy, shame, and ignorance that still veil this natural transition have carried over from the Victorian age with very little mitigation of the punishing stereotypes. "Menopause in the nineteenth century was described only in terms of what women lose at this stage of life," says Marilyn Yalom, senior scholar at the Stanford

University Institute for Research on Women and Gender. The Victorians were obsessed with women as reproductive creatures. Once barren and widowed, as they were likely to be by fifty, they were cued to view menopause as "the gateway to old age through which a woman passed at the peril of her life." Yalom's chapter in the documentary text *Victorian Women* quotes nineteenth-century obstetricians who taught that "the change of life unhinges the female nervous system and deprives women of their personal charm."

These attitudes were tempered somewhat by the sassy and energetic social activists who emerged between 1890 and 1920, a period that celebrated "the renaissance of the middle-aged." As death in childbirth was reduced, middle-class women began to appreciate the possibilities of a full life cycle and to cluster their childbearing in the earlier years of marriage. In their mature years they took up social causes, marched in parades, and founded movements. The great feminist leaders such as Elizabeth Cady Stanton celebrated the liberation of being in their fifties and continued as activists well into their sixties. *Cosmopolitan* magazine sang the praises of vital women of menopausal age in 1903: "The woman of fifty who only a few years ago would have been sent to the ranks of dowagers and grandmothers, today is celebrated for distinctive charm and beauty, ripe views, disciplined intellect, cultivated and manifold gifts." Once the Twenties got under way, however, the former stereotypes resurfaced.

The most famed and prolific women writers over the past hundred years have largely ignored, or been ignorant of, menopause. The romantic novels of George Sand, one of the most staggeringly prolific writers of the nineteenth

century in the French language, were read as widely as
Balzac's and Hugo's throughout the European continent.
Sand also penned twenty-five volumes of letters while
inspiring the music of her younger lover, Frédéric Cho-
pin. Yet in this vast landscape of words Marilyn Yalom
has uncovered only two personal letters in which Sand
refers to the symptoms of menopause. In the first, written to her editor, Hetzel, in 1853, Sand was forty-nine
years old:

> I am as well as I can be, given the crisis of my
> age. So far everything has taken place without
> grave consequence, but with sweats that I find
> overwhelming, and which are laughable be-
> cause they are imaginary. I experience the
> phenomenon of believing that I am sweating
> 15 or 20 times a day and night. . . . I have both
> the heat and the fatigue. I wipe my face with
> a white handkerchief and it is laughable be-
> cause I am not sweating at all. However, that
> makes me very tired.

Sand was chiding herself out of ignorance for having
hot flashes and night sweats. Often a woman does not
perspire, even though she is experiencing an abrupt leap
in skin temperature of one or two degrees. "Even today
it's very difficult to explain to a woman that it's a real
neurophysiological event, not a psychological event at all,
and therefore nothing she should be ashamed of," says
Dr. Robert Lindsay, an endocrinologist and leading researcher in the field of menopausal medicine at the Helen
Hayes Bone Center in West Haverstraw, New York. Not
until the mid-1970s were laboratory tests developed that

could demonstrate objectively the neurological discharge in the brain that causes the subjective changes women describe. When a woman says, "I am now having a hot flash," a machine similar to an EKG will show a spike in the ink line running across it.

George Sand refused to allow this inconvenience to interrupt her productivity and finished her letter by saying, "Nonetheless I am working and I've just done a play in three acts. . . ." Weeks later she indicated in a letter to her son that she had "rounded the horn" and felt better than she had for a long time. Sand was smart enough to know that even she should make a healthy adaptation in the exhausting nocturnal work habits she had devised, as a young mother, to work around domestic duties. "I sleep well, I eat well, I no longer have those flashes and I'm working without fatigue. It is true that I don't give myself to excess anymore and at one o'clock in the morning I wrap myself in my bed without hesitation."

One in the morning, for George Sand, was early. After fifty she stopped writing from midnight to 4:00 A.M. But by then she was a polished professional with twenty years of writing behind her, and she was able to ensconce herself at her country estate and produce the many novels for which she is famous. George Sand was still vibrant, and still writing, when she died at the age of seventy-two.

Anaïs Nin, another fearless watchwoman over the back alleys of the female psyche, neglected the subject in her writings. Virginia Woolf's fragile nature was bedeviled by physical illness and mental anguish at every stage. She attracted particularly harsh criticism for the book that expressed her viewpoint as a woman in her fifties, *Three*

Guineas. Woolf attributed none of her ills to menopause and never mentioned it in her writings, though she must have passed through it before she took her own life at fifty-nine. Colette was one of the rare writers to mention menopause at all in her work, portraying it in her novel *Break of Day* as both daunting and potentially empowering.

Patriarchal and primitive societies have done their part in prescribing the menstrual taboo. Just as they have fostered a division of women into two dimensions—good little ovulating wife, who is the passive receptacle, and the scarlet woman or witch, who is active, sexually dynamic, and terrifying—men in traditional cultures have isolated the menstruating woman as "unclean," "polluting," and "dangerous." One would logically think that the woman who is finished with the fearsome business of monthly bleeding would become better accepted, and in some traditional subcultures she is. But there is a new, subjective fear, and not just in primitive societies.

Middle-aged men, as they themselves begin to slow down, have a good deal of fear and envy of the physical, mental, sexual, and spiritual energies of fully evolved women—women who are beyond being objects defined by the male gaze and now fully conscious keepers of their own bodies. That fear is projected back onto women, causing us to wonder if we really are over the hill when we no longer have value primarily as erotic objects and reliable breeders.

D O C T O R S   S T I L L   I N
T H E   D A R K   A G E S

So often women say, "I'm waiting for my doctor to tell me what to do." Lamentably, few doctors are well informed about menopause, and many assume that the vaguely described symptoms are psychological in nature. Since physicians are temperamentally disposed to helping people, they, too, feel frustrated at the state of scientific ignorance about women's health in the middle years.

"You don't need to know about that yet" is one standard answer women are given. The doctor pats her on the head, and out the door she goes with her migrainous headaches, ill-defined blues, or unexplained fatigue— what could it be? More commonly, she won't even bring up menopause, and her gynecologist won't either. Some women spend the next three or five years making the rounds of internists, neurologists, even psychiatrists, with no resolution, because they all ignore the obvious.

The experience of a busy professional political activist in Washington is emblematic. Noticing her periods were scanty and intermittent, and feeling uncharacteristically draggy, she went to her internist and plunked down three hundred dollars for a complete physical. She was forty-nine. The physician took a considerable amount of blood for tests. The results shed no light on her condition. Only when the activist talked to a woman friend who asked, "What about your estrogen level?" did the light bulb flash on. She realized her doctor had not taken any hormone levels. He had never even mentioned menopause.

"The most important change going on in the body of a forty-nine-year-old woman was never addressed," she says, chagrined at her own passivity. "Doctors treat our bodies as though we're the same machines as men, and we're not."

Gynecologists by and large find the menopausal woman an unappealing patient. She isn't going to have any more babies. Apart from a hysterectomy, there is little chance she will require surgery—the moneymaking part of the practice—but she can be expected to complain about vague symptoms and ask questions for which even the sympathetic physician has only unsatisfactory answers. With candor, a dedicated female gynecologist describes the attitudes of many of her male colleagues: "They find us tedious because we're going to take up their time, and threatening because we're smart and we're grown-ups—we don't want any of their bullshit."

This is not to imply that all male gynecologists are dismissive or that all female gynecologists are sympathetic. Women who have felt the necessity to deny their femaleness in order to "pass" in male-dominated medical schools and hospital settings may disassociate from menopause entirely, and they can be quite brutal with women patients who bring them a grab-bag of complaints.

The busy doctor of either sex is likely to take an incomplete family history of the factors that impinge on menopause. Just how cursory these conversations can be is illustrated by the experience of a well-known columnist and her sister, both hard on age fifty. They consulted the same gynecologist in the Boston area to ask what to do. Despite their genetic likeness, one was told she was a good candidate for hormones. Her sister was cautioned not to take hormones. It turns out that the sisters had emphasized different subjective fears.

Dr. Mathilde Krim, the indefatigable AIDS activist and former pioneer in interferon research, relates another typical story. "Very early on in my life I was shocked by the great indifference of male doctors to the health problems particular to women," she says, recalling the unnecessary secondary suffering of a woman cancer patient at Memorial Sloan-Kettering. Dr. Krim had been called into the group of male physicians discussing the woman's case; her cancer was of the lung. The patient was asked what other medications she took. "Estrogen," she volunteered.

"That's the first thing to cut out," the men ordered.

"Why, if it makes her feel better?" demanded Dr. Krim. "It was absurd. The poor woman had all these problems with her lung cancer, and now she had to suffer hot flashes on top of it." But the male physicians were gratuitously adamant. And of course, the patient did not dare to raise a complaint.

More and more, however, educated women are beginning to see themselves as selective consumers of health care and refusing to accept the gynecologist's word as oracular. And when they find out how little the doctors know, or anybody knows, about this oldest of female physical transitions, they are mad as hell.

The TV producer mentioned earlier who suffered embarrassment with hot flashes at a dinner party is a case in point. When she reported her problem to her gynecologist, he said, noticeably bored, "Oh, yeah, fifty years old, you're right on target. Menopause."

"What can I do about it?" inquired the take-charge

producer, accustomed to handling an eight-million-dollar budget.

"You just start taking estrogen."

She asked what were the implications of taking hormones.

"Well, you'll have to go for a breast X-ray twice a year instead of once a year. But there's no risk."

"If there's no risk, then why do I have to go twice as often?" she replied, thinking logically. He brushed off her question with a few remarks that sounded as if he were reading out of a manual: *How to Handle the Over-the-Hill Patient.*

"That made me defiant," says the producer. Finally she insisted he tell her if there was anything that would treat the hot flashes. He told her about the old standby called Bellergal. He warned, "But that won't help with irritability, depression, crying—all the rest of it."

"Maybe I won't have any 'rest of it,' " the producer said, her adrenaline pumping full strength. "In the meantime, so I don't have to spend the next ten years in a terrycloth robe, I'll try the Bellergal." She got up to leave.

"You can do that," said the gynecologist, with what she read as an arrogant smirk. "But you'll be back."

The normal preamble to menopause is sometimes treated with a casualness bordering on the criminal. "This uterus looks a little bit tired," a male gynecologist told a forty-year-old North Carolina woman, "guess we'll take her out." It was typical of the attitude among some doctors that the uterus is little more than a nuisance. Since this patient was a housekeeper, without all the fancy scientific words to defend the tired "her," all she could do was "fight to keep my uterus."

At a higher status level, another southern woman, a fifty-three-year-old graduate student I will call Katherine, ran into a more subtle insensitivity from her male gynecologist and her male internist. Katherine had spent fifty years doing what she was "supposed" to do: fitting her life into the interstices of her children's and husband's lives. Once her children were well launched, Katherine felt a deep need to be "credentialed" as a professional. "But we're out of sync with the family life cycle," she observed. Determined to make up for lost time, she became accustomed to working seventeen hours a day to get her master's degree and apply for a doctoral program.

"Suddenly, passing fifty, I could barely function. I couldn't write a paper after four in the afternoon, but all my complaints were vague," she confessed. "Neither doctor would give me hormones. All they know is I'm not *supposed* to be trying to get my doctorate at fifty-three. Why don't I just go home and calm down?"

At some level we *know* when the Change begins to come upon us. The sense of unease or disequilibrium is something women feel, though it remains incomprehensible to those who have not experienced it. Isn't it amazing that women should allow organized medicine, filtered through a male perspective, to tell us how we feel? (How many men know what it's like to be one week late? Or two weeks early while you're teaching a class in a white suit?) Medical breakthroughs in this century have given us the gift of greatly extended life spans; now attention should be turned to bringing *healthier* life spans. And that means women must become informed, active consumers of good health care. But because up to the present day we have accepted a way of thinking that denies or denigrates this epic change in our bodies and the exciting new vistas it can open in our minds, we have failed to demand that decent scientific research be done.

Our tax dollars have supported massive research on heart disease among men (while leaving women out of those clinical trials entirely), but our national health institutes cannot give us any definitive data about the long-term impact of the body's post-reproductive state on women's health. The National Institutes of Health has spared only 13 percent of its revenues to study women's health. If you compare the level of our scientific knowledge about the causes and effects of menopause with the evolution of modern medicine, it is as though bacteria have not been discovered yet and we are still dependent on leeches and roots and shamans to cure what ails us.

Medical schools still use terms such as *the weeping of the uterus* to describe menstruation, assigning emotions to a bodily organ because it wasn't fertilized by male sperm that month. The classical medical terminology for menopause is *ovarian failure*.

Another way of seeing it would be as *ovarian fulfillment*. One has put in thirty or forty years of ripening eggs and enduring the hormonal mischief of monthly cycles, on the chance that a child is wanted. Enough, say most women in middle age. We're ready to move on now, to find our place in the world, free of the responsibilities of our procreative years. It's time to take risks and pursue passions and allow ourselves adventures perhaps set aside way back at thirteen, when we accepted the cultural script for our gender that ordinarily denied those dreams. It's time to play! And kick up some dust!

Menopause is no longer a marker that means "This

Way to the End." Today fifty is the apex of the female life cycle. And today menopause is more properly seen as the gateway to a Second Adulthood, a series of stages never before part of the predictable life cycle for other than the very long-lived.

If forty-five is the old age of youth, fifty is the youth of this Second Adulthood. In fact, we have roughly the same number of years to look forward to as we have already lived as reproductive women. You don't believe it, do you? Consider. Most women begin menstruating at about thirteen and begin stopping at around forty-eight—remaining defined, and confined, to some degree by their procreative abilities for thirty-five years. The life expectancy of a woman fortunate enough to live to age fifty is now eighty-one. So from the time she reaches perimenopause the average woman has thirty-three more years.

It is time to render normalcy to a normal physical process that ushers in the youth of our Second Adulthood. This is a passage as momentous as the rite of passage into adolescence. Indeed, the menopausal passage is almost the mirror image of the transition to adolescence for females, and it will take just as many years. Jolted into menstruating at twelve or thirteen—remember?— we needed five years or more for our bodies to adjust to our uniquely altered chemistry, while our minds struggled to incorporate our new self-image. So, too, must we readjust to *not* menstruating.

Just as we were apprehensive as eleven-year-olds, standing on the doorsill of childhood about to be pushed out into the unknown turbulence of puberty, so are we naturally nervous when approaching menopause about letting go of aspects of femininity that have defined us.

We become more acutely aware of health, appearance, economic security, and the harbingers of mortality.

C I N D E R E L L A

H I T S   M E N O P A U S E

As the pacesetters among baby boom–generation women discover menopause on their horizon, they will bring it out of the closet. It has been happening only in the last year, beginning with conversations that in a previous generation would have been unimaginable.

I went to Los Angeles to join in such conversations. It seems that my article had stirred up a little *frisson* of fright among some of the movers and shakers in the film community. In that world, where leading ladies never look a day over twenty-nine and studio executives start subtracting years from their résumés before they hit thirty, Hollywood producer Lynda Guber had picked up a copy of *Vanity Fair* and discovered a cloud on the horizon of her perfect existence.

"*Menopause!*" she shrieked. "God, I've never seen that word written."

Lynda is a sizzling redhead from Brooklyn who has reached the pinnacle of Hollywood society together with her husband, Peter Guber, producer of *Batman* and *Rain Man* and now the head of SONY Pictures Entertainment. The next day she bumped into Joanna Poitier at a Beverly Hills bistro and asked innocently, "How are you doing?"

"I'm a lunatic, I'm going through menopause and

empty nest at the same time," said the beautiful actress-wife of actor Sidney Poitier. (It is culture-specific to Hollywood to identify women by their husbands' professional status.)

This is fantastic, thought Lynda. *This woman is ready to talk about how she feels.* Lynda herself had already decided "the impact of menopause will not be devastating on me, that's what my holistic belief system tells me," but all she knew about it, in fact, was that the subject was a real no-no. Lynda is committed to being a consciousness-raiser of people in the movie business, having cofounded an organization, Education 1st!, that spreads positive messages through TV shows. She passed the word to a friend, Annie Gilbar, editor of *LA Style*. "Annie, I have an idea. I'd like to have a meeting on menopause with the girls." The first invitees backed off. But word spread, and before long it became such a cachet event there had to be a luncheon and a dinner group. I was invited to come out and speak to both. My friend and gynecologist, Dr. Patricia Allen, accompanied me.

Going to Hollywood to talk about menopause was a little bit like going to Las Vegas to sell savings accounts. Such is the fetish of youthfulness in Southern California, one half expects there to be an ordinance against menopause there. "Women who are menopausal in California are around the bend—they view it like cancer," I was warned by a Chinese medicine specialist with a deluxe and desperate clientele in Los Angeles.

Nevertheless, it was a golden opportunity. California women in the boomer vanguard are normally the most uninhibited among their species in speaking out about whatever bothers them. I quickly discovered, however, that even they—women who have access to the most up-to-date information, women who are religious about doing the stations of their Nautilus machines, women who have phone indexes of dozens of doctors, not to mention the best acupuncturists, herbalists, liposuctionists, and shrinks—*even they* didn't have any answers on menopause. In fact, they had never discussed the questions, even among themselves. When they did come together to confront the subject, they reflected many of the secret fears and defensive reactions common among women everywhere.

Lynda invited us to gather at her Japanese-style fantasy beach house. At the door each woman was invited to leave her shoes on a shelf and choose a kimono. I kept looking for a gray hair in the crowd—scarcely a one among this mostly blond, mid-fortyish group. The guests draped themselves over big black cushions on tansu boxes in the screening room. It was reminiscent of slumber parties in junior high, when girls played dress-up and talked about taboo subjects like sex. But now we were grownups; and the very fact these prominent women had showed up, in this subculture, was an act of bravery.

"I invited Glenn Close to come," said one of the women. "I thought she was going to faint dead away."

I began by asking those present to introduce themselves, give their age, and say why they had come—what meaning did menopause have for them? The wife of one of the town's top studio executives confessed she usually shunned "negative subjects," but her mother was dead, and she had no one else to consult. A woman who heads her own company described herself as an information junkie. "My gynecologist tells me that I'm not going through the Change at all, but I know my body, and I feel different over the past year. I've had occasional night sweats. I used to think I had a virus."

Lisa Specht, a lawyer who appears as the legal correspondent on ABC-TV's *Home Show*, has no children and said she didn't think she had to worry about menopause, at least until she was fifty-five or something. "I haven't had any symptoms yet, except that my skin has been oily," she assured herself.

The outspoken Joanna Poitier broke the ice. She was willing to admit she might be going through menopause, although her primary concern was letting go of her two daughters, now eighteen and twenty. "I keep waking up in the middle of the night, changing my nightgown. I went to the gynecologist, and she told me that I was still moist. She said I won't probably go into menopause for another two years. I have night sweats. I tried it without the duvet and the nightgown, and I still have night sweats. I have day sweats, too! The back of my neck is damp all day long."

The next speaker was immediately recognizable. Lesley Ann Warren, the movie actress we all remember from her ethereal portrayal of Cinderella in the TV musical, is even more beautiful today. Her features are still delicate, her body is still slim and supple, and reddish brown hair ripples over her shoulders. More appealing than all that are the quickened intelligence and candor that she has earned over forty years and has brought to her more recent roles in the films *Victor/Victoria* and *Choose Me*. But Lesley Ann makes her living here in Cinderella Land, where girls are never supposed to grow up. Hollywood ruthlessly cuts the finest actresses once they reach forty—

yes, even Meryl! Studio executives will callously describe a thirty-eight-year-old actress who is still gorgeous as "over the hill" or "She's an old hag." As an actress in that workplace, Lesley Ann Warren is torn between her liberated feminist beliefs and the devastating reality that every day her worth is judged by her age and her looks.

Divorced from Jon Peters, former co-head of the former Columbia Studios, with whom she had a son, Lesley Ann has been single for some time. She now has a new love. It was he who found a photocopy of my *Vanity Fair* article lying around. Lesley Ann wanted to educate herself on the subject before it happened so she could deal with it homeopathically and herbally, as she does everything else. She had forgotten to hide the evidence.

"You know, I read this article," he said casually one night.

Omigod, he's found me out! was the actress's first thought. "I was really scared he would think *I* was menopausal. I felt ashamed." But he surprised her.

"I'm glad I read it. I feel like any man who's in a relationship with a woman dealing with this must be very loving, very aware, and very present," he said.

Lesley Ann counted her new love among an ultramicroscopic subspecies of the male genus, at least as it is bred by the movie business. "In all the rest of my experience, men are so staggeringly uneducated in this area, it's deadly for us," she told the group. "Most men I know run from the word *menopause*."

"We're afraid to educate the men, that's our problem," amended Joanna. "I have never been afraid to say how old I am. I've never had surgery or collagen or anything like that. And I don't feel any less terrific because I'm menopausal. Whoever you are with, they should experience the whole thing that you're experiencing." Joanna added vociferously, "I take no aspirin, no Tylenol; if I have a headache, I live through it. I don't believe in pills. I know that I will not take hormones, because to me it's unnatural."

The word *holistic* was almost a fetish in this group. Used indiscriminately, it might be intended to mean one who never uses Tylenol, or one who has stopped taking drugs and alcohol, or one who consults Chinese medical doctors and herbalists but *never* a member of the AMA. A bouncy talent agent with a blond boy-cut admitted she was taking hormones; *admitted*, because, like so many women, her decision was tinged with guilt. "I knew something was up when I went to a restaurant and had to ask the waiter for two menus—one to see what I was ordering and the other to fan myself."

Knowing laughter rippled through the group. We decided that if we met again, we would call ourselves The Fan Club.

The agent revealed a more intimate reason for her decision. "One night when my husband and I were having sex, it felt like I was a virgin. I said, 'Something is wrong here.' My gynecologist took a blood test and told me it was the Change of Life." She emphasized that she was on a very low dose of hormone replacement therapy and that she was happy with the results.

Joanna Poitier broke in with a question on everybody's mind. "Is it okay to go through the rest of life without estrogen?"

Dr. Allen said there was no definitive answer. "When

we are in this part of our lives, we have to make decisions about what it is that we want. Beyond the symptomatic discomforts, there are also medical issues that bear on our long-term health—osteoporosis, heart disease, breast and uterine cancer." Dr. Allen's advice was to gather as much information as possible, including that concerning one's own family history, to find out if there is a medical reason to take hormone replacement therapy, and then make a decision.

"But we don't have to make a decision for life. We make a decision for three months, and then we make a decision again," she added, sowing visible relief in some of the tense faces. Others were impatient with this answer. They had come looking for a risk-free, all-natural curative.

Mary Miccuci introduced herself as a "stress queen." A tall, Cher-like streak of a woman who started her own catering business, Along Came Mary, she dashes around Hollywood putting on spreads for the stars. Her signs of menopause began with palpitations; she thought she was having a heart attack. "The quality of my life is changing—all of our lives are changing. I want information!" she said angrily, pitching forward to lean her elbows on her knees. "I want to go through this process as quickly as possible. I'm on a holistic journey to deal with it. Are there the right herbs to take care of the silent killers—heart disease and osteoporosis?"

Surely what they all wanted to hear from me and Dr. Allen was that some magic regimen—yoga and yogurt, or yams and ginseng and green leafy vegetables—would allow them to remain as middle-aged women exactly as they had been: youthful wives, sexually appealing and responsive lovers, efficient career builders. They were not yet ready to consider a new self-definition. And until one is ready, the information that is available is not much use.

"I think that we have all been too passive about what the outcome of our lives should be," Mary continued huffily. "Because I tell you, the way I felt for a year was pretty shitty. I have a five-and-a-half-year-old little girl, and I want to be so together for this kid. This menopause stuff, I'll be goddamned if I'll let it get in my way."

Mary's hostility toward the whole subject was revelatory. She had become used to managing her life like a man, according to goals, timetables, balance sheets. She is a businesswoman accustomed to efficiency; in fact, she had to leave early to cater a screening party for Bette Midler's latest film. But now, at the peak of her productivity, she is feeling violated by this reassertion of her body's biologic identity. There is nothing efficient about "this menopause stuff."

Aloma Ichinose, a photographer equally active in her career, had taken the opposite approach. "I'm going through the Change right now. I feel great about it. But at first it was a nightmare. I was raised by a man, so none of this was ever talked about." Allowing time for trial and error, Aloma had made several different decisions over the previous year. When urine and blood tests confirmed that she was in menopause, her doctor put her on Premarin. To her, it felt like doing drugs. "I did the Premarin for six months. I felt wonderful, and all my symptoms—the disrupted sleep, the forgetfulness—went away." She added defensively, "I'm not into drugs. I haven't had a drink in years. But I was really worried about bone loss. I'm active, I'm a photographer, I need my strength." Eventually the fear and guilt over taking hormones got to her, and after the six months she stopped. "And all the symptoms returned," she admitted. "I just didn't feel well, and so I'm back on it again and I feel good."

An art gallery owner pressed the issue of age prevention. "How long do you take this? Will it prolong our youth? We are young in our forties, where people of other generations weren't. I'm forty-seven years old, but I don't think that I am forty-seven in numbers. I have the same energy as always."

Joanna, whose blond tendrils and soft curves help her to maintain the jolly all-American-girl good looks of a perpetual cheerleader, is able to maintain the illusion of her inner eye: "I still feel like I'm twenty-eight. I wear my hair the same way, I'm twenty-eight years old."

Another woman in the room muttered, "But you're not. And they *know* you're not."

It cut like a flesh wound into the self-image of every woman there. They were all attractive, and that statement didn't even need the qualifying prefix *still*. External beauty wasn't the real problem. It was the dysynchrony between their idealized inner images—the women they were at their nubile peaks—and blanks where the faces and bodies and spirits of their future selves would have to be filled in, sooner or later. As vanguard baby boomers they agreed, they belonged to the most pampered, narcissistic, and obstinately adolescent generation in American history. "We have delayed duty, responsibility and commitment," wrote a spokeswoman for their generation, Lynn Smith, in the *Los Angeles Times*. "We have dieted, jogged, and exercised so much we look and actually *think* we are five to ten years younger than we are."

The most telling reaction of all came from a sleek-looking South African woman who had been mute all night. Before I left, she took me aside and asked the quintessential Southern California question: "Tell me, what can I do so I *don't have to have this?*"

BOOMERS'
GIFT TO WOMEN

As a woman looks ahead to the Change, it is natural to focus entirely on the loss of powers one has taken for granted in previous stages. The youthful looks you could always trade on, and the magical powers of procreation that connected you to the cycle of all life—these are the God-given, gloriously unfair advantages of being born a well-formed woman. Suddenly, in the mid-forties, one must face the fact that these powers are ebbing. What will replace them?

The women who attended the luncheon meeting in Beverly Hills were ready to confront such issues. They were a mix of professionals who had left a mark on their respective fields: A top state politician, a mayor, and a judge were interspersed with well-known screenwriters, entertainment producers, and social activists. All but three of those present were in their mid-forties with still-young children.

"So many of us know each other," Annie Gilbar kept

remarking, "and we talk about a lot of things—children, sex, everything—but this subject has never come up. Not once." Two of the creative talents in today's film industry were among the group: Meg Kasdan, co-screenwriter with husband Lawrence Kasdan of *Grand Canyon*, and executive producer Carole Isenberg (*The Color Purple* and *This Is My Life*). Both were flabbergasted when they couldn't think of a single reference in a film to a woman going through the Change and the impact it had on her life. "I'm always sneaking messages in about women's lives, but never this," said Carole. "It's a sorry statement that shows how unwilling and uncomfortable we have been to deal with this issue." Meg added, "Mature women—that is, over forty—are almost invisible in Hollywood movies."

Once people began to talk about menopause as more than a matter of spigots and pipes and secretions involving our organs, an important issue surfaced. Losing the magic—that was the deeper mutation to be accepted. The graduation from our fertile years resonates in our psyches as deeply as the squirm and throb in the belly of our first pregnancy signify our awesome powers of creation. Like most graduations, it is the occasion for both relief and sadness.

"For many of us who waited until we were well into our thirties and even early forties before having children, the physical power of giving birth is still palpable; it touches something very deep and instinctual," ventured Suzanne Rosenblatt Buhai, a psychotherapist. "That flame of the instinctual being extinguished is not as readily dealt with as one might think."

Dealing with loss is one of the tasks we struggle with

in every passage, but it is particularly poignant as women notice the first skips in a fertility we have probably taken for granted. The feelings were brought out by a woman who has obviously delighted in maternity. Joyce Bogart Trabulus has two children and a quartet of stepchildren in her life and is further fulfilled by community caretaking in the form of running charities for cancer and AIDS research. She has no desire to have any more children. No *daylight world* desire.

"And yet I really feel sadness every time I think about it," she admitted. "I was forty-one when I had my last child, who's three years old now—I almost feel like a grandmother to my own kid. And I sometimes catch myself thinking, *Oh, God, this is fabulous, I'd love to do this again.* It's a great loss to know that it will be impossible for me. It's not like I want another one. And I'm not menopausal, or even pre-menopausal. But I look at a baby and say, 'Oh.' "

Suzanne mused out loud, "Given our generational narcissism—whether it's because of our sheer numbers, Dr. Spock, or the dominant influence of psychoanalysis —I just wonder if this concern with self is now being focused on menopause. Are we getting all worked up over something that is, in fact, quite normal and has been experienced since time immemorial? Perhaps the best gift we can give society at this stage is to see this as something very positive. If we can normalize this experience, as Gail says, it will help women deal with it. Otherwise, women will take on the responsibility of this somehow being their fault—they are supposed to be pulling out of this funk."

One of the few women in the room over fifty, Vicki

Reynolds, mayor of Beverly Hills, looked around the group with eagerness and some envy. "I am almost a generation ahead of most of you," she said. "I have seen women my age go through menopause without the benefit of any medical enlightenment—ignorant of all you have been saying. Now we look to you, the baby boom generation, to talk about this openly and explore the effects and benefits of menopause. That's so exciting."

It was agreed that the vestigial attitude surrounding menopause—"I'm no good anymore"—would be changed by the way women like themselves handled it. I suggested, only half seriously, "If every woman in menopause told five people in the next week, those five people would have an entirely different view of it. 'This dish is in menopause? Well, maybe it isn't so terrible.' "

Dr. Allen observed that at this stage we have responsibilities to the world, not just to our communities. She is excited every day by finding new channels to educate women about their bodies. "That's my public passion," she said. "But we also need something for ourselves—new passions all the time."

I added wickedly, "And they may include a twenty-five-year-old lover."

"Yeah, a *blind* twenty-five-year-old lover!" amended one of the California women.

With a whooping and shimmying of laughter, the session ended. Seventeen women went out into the world to resume their balancing acts among careers, husbands, children, car pools, social and spiritual lives, too busy to worry much about menopause, but better prepared for the future. Laughter and forgetting . . . two of the best gifts women of any age can share with one another.

But something hopeful, something even incendiary had come out of those two sessions with California women. Their need to know was beginning to overcome their fear of knowing. It convinced me that the pacesetting women of this generation will shift the boundaries as well as the meaning of menopause: They will redefine it, and *live it*, as a mid-life experience of minor importance in the scheme of a long and lushly various life.

ROSEANNE
IN   MENOPAUSE?

Many less privileged women assume that menopause is just another burden of being a woman and simply bear it, though not grinning. But the class differences are glaring. The population tapped for the rare studies has been almost exclusively white, well educated, and motivated to take care of its health preventively. The vast majority of women in lower socioeconomic groups have no idea of the long-term health issues related to "the Change." They are so accustomed to bleeding and having cramps and premenstrual tension that when they hit menopause they just shrug and say, "Here we go again—male doctors treating me like I don't matter a damn."

That was Kate McNally's first reaction. A secretarial assistant in local government in a medium-size Long Island town, she is now fifty-four. All her life Kate has been a great coper, having had four children close together and launched them all as young adults of whom she can be proud. Her reward? "The most frustrating phase I've ever been through in my life—it's horrendous! I've never felt so helpless. Nobody understands menopause. And nobody knows what to do about it."

Kate went to her gynecologist complaining of heavy bleeding. After a questionable Pap smear, a cone biopsy was done, followed by a D&C. She was put on estrogen and told to have a mammogram. The results weren't conveyed to her for two months. A lump had been found. Of course, at first she blamed the hormones. But the great majority of breast tumors, including hers, are slow-growing. Her disease had probably been developing, undetected, for several years. The irony is, many women do not bother with a mammogram *until* they consult a doctor about indications of menopause. If a tumor is found, the culprit may look like hormones but is probably the result of more careful medical surveillance.

After two lumpectomies, Kate is off estrogen forever and bedeviled by menopausal symptoms no one can tell her how to relieve. "I feel betrayed," she says softly. "I've always put others before myself. By this age I have more money to work with and more leisure time with the kids gone. I should have the energy to do the things I've always wanted." I asked what things she had looked forward to.

"Getting a decent night's sleep." This modest expectation is betrayed by the dull film over her blue eyes. "You go for years with little babies waking you up all night. Then the teen years, when you can't sleep for worrying because they're out in your car. And now *I'm* the one awake all night!" She laughs hard. Her husband seems wonderfully supportive, and Kate is determined to cope with this stage as she has with other trials in the past. But after months of sleep deprivation, no wonder Kate, like so many menopausal women, says she feels frustrated.

Her sister, Bindy, is only forty-two and very attractive, with long, curly red hair and a sugar-doughnut figure wrapped in shorts and a T-shirt, but already she is wrestling with the emotional preamble to menopause. "I used to be the no-worry type. Just leave the house, go to the beach—nothing ever bothered me," she says. "I lost my temper but once in a blue moon." Now she's a virtual powder keg. When her son didn't come to the table until his dinner was cold, she jumped up in such a childish rage she knocked over a chair. "Everybody looked at me as if I had three heads."

She told her girlfriend later, "They measured the chemicals in my brain with a blood test. They said the chemical was out of balance and that indicated I was in menopause."

"That explains why you're so moody," sympathized her friend.

"Moody! I'm not moody!" Bindy remembers shrieking. "How can you say that? You're my best friend!"

These powerful hormones do, in fact, cross the blood-brain bridge. Sensors in the brain that control emotions pick up a signal when there is an erratic production of either estrogen or progesterone. In a person whose nervous system is finely tuned, these sensors overreact, triggering brain-chemistry changes and emotional symptoms. Veteran gynecologists affirm that some women can have physical symptoms from even slight changes in the amount of estrogen produced.

Every morning, as a waitress in a busy coffee shop, Bindy has to stroke hundreds of people who haven't had coffee yet. "The doctor told me to stop smoking, cut down on cholesterol, and avoid stress. Ha, avoid stress! How?"

She knows she is being grouchy and impossible. "But I can't control it. And I'm afraid if I take this estrogen, then *I'll* have lumps like my sister."

ACROSS COLOR, CLASS, AND CULTURE LINES

The chief reason for the silence and apprehension surrounding the subject of menopause in American society is our phobia about aging. Cross-cultural studies of women and menopause reveal that the Change of Life is experienced differently depending on one's cultural assumptions about aging, femininity, and the societal role of the older woman. When the American sociologist Pauline Bart studied anthropological accounts of the status of women in a large number of cultures, she found that the feminine role assumed by a woman in her fertile years was in all cultures reversed after menopause.

Anthropologist Mary Catherine Bateson points out: "In many societies women are granted a greater degree of freedom after menopause than they were permitted in their reproductive years. This may be because women no longer represent a risk of 'pollution,' or no longer need to be sequestered as sex objects through whom their husbands might be dishonored." Indian women of the Rajput caste do not complain of depression or psychological symptoms of menopause since they are freed from veiled invisibility and at last are able to sit and joke with the men, reports anthropologist Marcha Flint. Furthermore, in some traditional societies, such as Iran's, women come into their own only when they have adult sons. Bateson describes how grown-up sons pay court to their mothers, visiting them with news and flowers.

Similarly, anthropologist Margaret Lock reports that 65 percent of Japanese women consider menopause uneventful. The Japanese language does not even have a word for hot flashes. (A report in *The Lancet*, however, describes "sinking spells" among Japanese women, rather like the swooning of Victorian women.) In China, where age is venerated, menopausal symptoms are rarely reported.

In fact, findings presented at the Sixth International Congress on the Menopause, held in Bangkok in late 1990, confirmed that women in Eastern countries report fewer and less severe symptoms than menopausal women in the West—even though the mean age was the same across the board (around fifty-one years). The study included women from Hong Kong, Malaysia, the Philippines, South Korea, Taiwan, Indonesia, and Singapore.

But in America youth and desirability go hand in hand, and the role for the older woman is uncertain at best. So, although menopause in the United States is defined primarily in hormonal terms, cultural attitudes cast the signs and symptoms in a negative light. Of twenty-five hundred Massachusetts women ages forty-five to fifty-five studied by Harvard sociologist John McKinlay and epidemiologist Sonja McKinlay, most anticipated menopause with relief. But for those whose self-worth rested primarily in appearance and sexual desirability, passing fifty was like *taking the veil*; suddenly they felt invisible.

Although I did not undertake a "scientific" sampling of American women's menopausal experiences, I did speak with over a hundred women from diverse racial, class, and educational backgrounds. I discovered that the women who enjoy a boost in postmenopausal status and self-esteem are those who perform roles in which intellect, judgment, creativity, or spiritual strength is primarily valued—politicians, educators, lawmakers, doctors, nurse supervisors, therapists, writers, artists, clergywomen, etc.—while women whose worth was earlier judged primarily on their looks and sex appeal—movie actresses, performers, many full-time wives and mothers—are diminished in status. We know that middle-class housewives who are over-involved with their children are the most likely to suffer depression in this stage of life. But they, too, are able to change stale self-images if they are willing to leave the comfort of familiarity and take the risk of starting a new direction in their Second Adulthood. Women who build close bonds to grandchildren may make themselves indispensable and often enjoy a tender and playful intimacy that brings them closer than they were to their own children.

African-American women in general are more likely than white women to pass through menopause with no psychological problems. One possible reason is the dominance of grandmothers in maintaining the extended black family; it is often granny who assumes a primary care role for offspring of her unmarried children. Also, osteoporosis is seldom a concern for women of color. However, they have their own physical vulnerability—fibroid tumors—a vulnerability often worsened by cultural attitudes.

Fibroids are benign growths found in 20 percent of all women. They are far more common among African-American women than white women, according to the National Black Women's Health Project. They often lead women to unnecessary hysterectomies. As a result, says Frances Dorey, chair of the project, "Black women are lucky if they even make it to menopause with a uterus." The medical reason they have a higher incidence of fibroids remains unknown (African-American women are generally excluded from the studies or are unidentified by race in clinical trials). It is not even known exactly how many hysterectomies are performed on women each year in the United States, because there is no organization that keeps national statistics on hysterectomies. In fact, the National Center for Health Statistics does not have a department that deals specifically with gynecological issues.

Pamela Pilate's job as a nurse with the giant California HMO Kaiser Permanente is to do menopause education. Many state employees and low-income women come to her classes in downtown Los Angeles. She holds two kinds of classes, and when I asked her if she had noticed any cultural differences in attitudes women bring in, Pilate said something startling even to herself:

"The white women attend my menopause class. The black and Hispanic women come to my hysterectomy class." Women of color or low income who present an assigned Medicaid doctor with symptoms common to the "fearsome forties"—heavy, clotted bleeding and cramps such as they haven't had since before bearing their children—are most likely to be steered toward a hysterectomy. By the time they are referred to a nurse-counselor like Pamela Pilate, they already have a date for surgery.

As an African-American woman herself Pilate is dismayed by how passively many of her patients approach this surrender of their reproductive organs. "When women of color have female problems, their usual reaction is to wait," she reports. "It's denial or fear." Lack of basic medical knowledge about their own bodies also plays a large part. As Pilate notes, "White women look for other alternatives—nutrition, herbs, or less invasive surgical procedures for removing the benign growths." By the time the black women come to her hysterectomy class, they have waited a long time to see a doctor, and they are either in pain or suffering from heavy bleeding or urinary problems. The fibroid may have grown to the size of a grapefruit. When Pilate inquires if their surgeon also plans to remove their ovaries, most of the women have no idea. "Usually they don't know the function of their ovaries."

Pilate's lecture stresses that hysterectomy is a last resort. She also emphasizes that as a woman approaches menopause, uterine fibroids usually shrink if she doesn't take hormone replacement therapy. "But the women I see have a cut-and-dried attitude. 'This is part of life, what else? Let's get it over with.'" The highest point of consciousness raising Pilate can usually orchestrate is to get the women to go back and ask, "Okay, Doctor, why do you think that my ovaries should go?"

In *Essence* magazine Dr. Ezra C. Davidson, Jr., president of the American College of Obstetricians and Gynecologists, confirmed Pilate's anecdotal observation: "By the time black women get into a doctor's office, their presentation of fibroid tumors is often dramatic."

"You're going to have a hysterectomy, just like my sister, cousin, mother, aunt, daughter, et cetera" was the message repeated like a folk belief to Marsha Carruthers of Grand Rapids, Michigan, when she consulted friends and physicians about her fibroids. A professional health consultant to women of color all over the country, Carruthers was adamant about avoiding this surgery. She read about barks and herbs said to be effective in reducing menstrual flow and benign tumors—white oak bark, slippery elm bark, witch hazel, etc. She took the herbs in capsules and altered her diet radically, cutting out red meat, sugar, white flour, and processed foods. Within a month her cycle regulated itself.

Although the popularity of hysterectomy is highest in the South—"Mississippi Appendectomy" it's called—and lowest in the Northeast, where statistically there are more educated women, a stylish ob-gyn man in Beverly Hills recommends "prophylactic hysterectomies" along with removal of the ovaries when a woman reaches menopause. His philosophy in advising this major surgical operation for a healthy woman is that it does away with the risks of uterine and ovarian cancer. While many hysterectomies are unnecessary, clear indicators do exist for hysterectomy in women with fibroid tumors: first, rapid growth of the tumor, which may be a sign of cancer developing in the fibroid; second, uncontrollable bleeding; third, fibroid size so large that other organs may be compromised; or, finally, intractable pain. It is estimated that only 11 percent of hysterectomies are performed to eliminate cancerous growths.

A Seattle divorcée brags about solving the whole dilemma by having just such a hysterectomy at the age of forty-one. "My doctor was a yanker instead of a saver," she quips. "But I wasn't going to use the equipment anymore; I didn't want it. I'm glad I got rid of my ovaries."

It may sound like a nice mid-life housecleaning, but in fact, removal of both ovaries is castration. Twice as many women who have hysterectomies today, compared with twenty years ago, also have their ovaries removed. It is common, and realistic, for a woman with a persistent ovarian tumor to have at least one ovary removed. However, when both ovaries are removed, the abrupt and total, rather than gradual, shutting down of ovarian function can be devastating, placing the woman at risk of serious depression. It also extinguishes sexual desire. And unless a woman immediately starts hormone replacement therapy and commits to remaining on the medication indefinitely, she will have all the symptoms of menopause, whatever her age. What's more, early surgical removal of the ovaries *doubles* the risk of osteoporosis. If you lose your ovaries at age thirty, by the time you reach age fifty, your *bone age* may be seventy. Yet doctors often refuse to warn a woman that the surgery can have such lifelong effects even after the body heals.

Another reason for the fear inspired by the prospect of menopause is the assumption that it takes place at a single point in time. "Women are very frightened that at age forty-nine, all these things they've read about—heart disease, osteoporosis, vaginal atrophy—will happen all at once," says Professor Phyllis Mansfield. "No distinction is made between women's lives at fifty and at seventy. We would never do this with men."

It is important, then, to distinguish among the various phases of the long menopausal passage. More changes probably take place during this passage than at any other time in a woman's adult life. And as one moves through the physical, psychological, social, and spiritual aspects of the transition, dramatic shifts in perspective occur. There may be a transformation in the sense of time, of self in relation to others, and a rethinking of the negative vs. positive aspects of moving into a new and unfamiliar state of being.

The acute period of biological passage, or ovarian transition, spans five to seven years—usually from forty-seven or forty-eight to the mid-fifties. But it is the beginning of a long and little-mapped stage of post-reproductive life. I propose three demarcations of this Second Adulthood for contemporary Western women: perimenopause (start of the transition); menopause (completion of the ovarian transition); and a stage I will call coalescence—the mirror image of adolescence—in which women can tap into the new vitality Margaret Mead called "postmenopausal zest."

The
Perimenopause
Panic

he earliest phase, perimenopause, is reminiscent of the first time one got one's period—the I-could-die feeling when a girlfriend whispered, "You have a spot on the back of your skirt," and you had to back out of the glee club rehearsal so no one would see. And now, at the dignified apex of one's adulthood, to have to worry about being hit with surprise periods, hot flashes, night sweats, insomnia, incontinence, sudden bouts of waistline bloat, heart palpitations, crying for no reason, temper outbursts, migraines, itchy, crawly skin, memory lapses—my God, what's going on?

It is during perimenopause—in their forties—that women feel most estranged from their bodies. The important thing to know is that for two to three years the female body is out of sync with its own chemistry.

Half of all women who have hot flashes will begin feeling them while they are still menstruating normally, starting as early as age forty. Studies show that most women have hot flashes for two years. One quarter of women have them for five years. And 10 percent have them for the rest of their lives.

The first sign of perimenopause, however, is very often *not* hot flashes but gushing: a sudden heavy flow of blood that may be dark or clotted and that may seep through the normal protection. Dr. Allen tells patients in their forties, "Your cycle will get longer or shorter, lighter or heavier, closer together or farther apart. This is all normal." She adds, "Almost everybody bleeds erratically during perimenopause."

(It happens when we stop ovulating every month. The months when ovulation doesn't occur, we produce no progesterone—the hormone ordinarily responsible for flushing the lining of the uterus. The endometrial lining becomes thicker and may not be entirely discarded until the next cycle, when the body deals with the previous buildup.)

One month a woman may have a heavy period, another month nothing; all of a sudden she may develop cysts in her breast, or functional ovarian cysts, and two months or a year later she may be back to normal. The reason for all the volatility is that hormone levels are surging and falling in frantic response to desperate signals from the brain to the pituitary. Her menstrual cycle not only becomes erratic but is uncoupled from her temperature and sleep cycles and affects her appetite, sexual interest, and overall sense of well-being. The body's whole balance is thrown off. While this can be very unsettling, it is *a temporary phenomenon*, and one should not be railroaded into a hysterectomy or onto hormones.

Phyllis Mansfield, the Penn State academic who spear-headed research on female cycles, registered the first signs of the Change in herself in her early forties. Having always had a normal and very predictable cycle, she was unnerved when her periods became heavier and more frequent. "I would have to schedule family camping trips and conferences around my cycle." Although she studied and went for checkups, still, in the back of her mind, was a common fear: *Are my organs deteriorating?*

She noticed something odd, too, about her moods. As a researcher she knew that premenstrual stress occurs after ovulation. But when one's cycle becomes erratic, with periods every two or three weeks, or two or three months apart, how does one know when, or if, ovulation occurs?

"I'd have a really long period of magnificent energy and acute mental functioning, even brilliance, when I was never tired, always very up, producing like crazy. At first I thought, *Oh! So this is going to be part of my new personality*. Then just as suddenly I fell into a period of intense anxiety—and that lasted for a month. I thought, *So, is this it?* But once I got my period, the despond just lifted and dissipated in one day. So then you think, *What happens when there are no more cycles? Is there one mood that persists? Is it permanent mellowing? Permanent anything?*"

What happens if I can't be me anymore?

Erratic hormone activity may play mischief with a woman's equilibrium in any one of dozens of ways. Ruth Jacobowitz, co-author with gynecologist Wulf Utian of *Managing Your Menopause*, describes a perimenopause of several years of episodes in which "I was shaking but you couldn't see it. I would hold out my hand, it would be perfectly still, but inside there was an electrical sensation of my heart beating too fast. Turns out, it was palpitations, and palpitations are one symptom of estrogen loss."

Some women have all the indicators, some none; it is highly individual, and somewhat subjective, so that when one woman turns to another for advice, the likelihood is she will pass on misinformation. The vast majority of women have no idea they are in something called "perimenopause." Yet a woman's attitude and awareness going into this momentous passage have a profound impact on how it is experienced. As we know, the last person most women consult for information is a doctor. Those who do have often reached the point of panic.

"I think I'm going crazy" is a frequent frightened admission Dr. Morris Notelovitz hears at the Women's Health Center in Gainesville, Florida. "Many women feel it's very difficult to concentrate. They can hear what's going on, they know they're there, but it's as though their body is just witnessing." These are the women whose hormones are falling and spiking and falling again, six times a day or even a half dozen times within an hour. They feel—and, in fact, they are—out of control of their bodies. They may also feel at the mercy of erratic moods. Is it all in their minds?

DANCING

AROUND

DEPRESSION

Whether or not depression is associated with menopause has been a subject of intense debate, mostly because of a looseness of terminology and perhaps subjective fears on the part of some researchers. The much-publicized Massachusetts Women's Health Study reported in a 1986 Harvard Medical School publication that "depression in middle-aged women is associated mainly with events and circumstances unrelated to the hormonal changes that occur at menopause." Epidemiologist Sonja McKinlay, co-author of the study with her husband, John, insisted in an interview: "Most women just go straight through menopause, no problem. None, nor with irritability."

Try out that line on a room full of menopausal-aged women and one is guaranteed a laugh. The McKinlays' conclusion—that depression at this stage is associated *only* with external "social circumstances"—was suspect since it was a paper-and-pencil questionnaire and no measurements had been taken of the actual hormone levels in peri- and postmenopausal women.

Of the many stories I had been told by women themselves, a typical description of menopausal malaise came from a woman I'll call Nora. A former tavern owner, she was remarried as she started her forties and had happily moved to the country. She had never been depressed before. At forty-six, when she began skipping periods, a fog of indeterminate sadness came over her from out of left field.

"I'd go out and walk for five miles every morning on a country road, sun shining, birds singing—and tears would start running down my cheeks. Why? I kept looking at my life—was there anything to validate this depression?" she recalled asking. "Nothing. I was normally very up. My doctor told me I was too young for menopause. Then I remembered times in adolescence when I'd come home from school, go into my room, sit down on my bed, and cry. That's when I knew. Whatever these doctors say, it's my hormones." Her malaise, although frightening at the time, lifted within several months.

It is true that *clinical* depression subsides in women over fifty. And irritability and depression in middle-aged women do have many other sources. But mood changes are so commonly mentioned by women in the perimenopause phase, why should women be told there is no hormonal basis for feeling depressed?

"That's looking at major depression as a disease," stresses Dr. Howard Fillit, a gerontologist at Mount Sinai Hospital in New York City. "A woman comes into a doctor's office at age fifty-one with the menopause and says, 'Doctor, I can't function very well in the office. I think I have memory loss, I can't pay attention to my work, and I feel really depressed.' If the doctor reads the literature, he knows that there's no major association of depression with the menopause, so he says, 'C'mon, you're crazy.' If the doctor was aware that these complaints and symptoms are real, although they may not qualify as a disease, this problem could be dealt with in a constructive manner."

Up to 80 percent of menopausal women in self-report studies describe feeling nervousness and irritability.

In fact, estrogen does improve mood and the sense of psychological well-being even in well-adjusted women who have no distressing menopausal symptoms, according to a brand-new study done by Dr. Edward Ditkoff at the University of Southern California School of Medicine. Women in the random study who were given the standard dose of 0.625 mg of estrogen a day showed a decided improvement in depression scores and were more optimistic and confident than those given placebos. Neurobiologically estrogen has chemical effects on the brain similar to those of antidepressants. The most experienced researchers say that when estrogen levels in the blood are very low, a woman might start to feel a bit sad or blue or notice irritability or mood swings, but not of a clinical magnitude.

That is the key distinction: Women low in estrogen often have feelings of malaise, as opposed to suffering from the *DSM-III* criteria of depression as disease (the criteria used in the McKinlays' Massachusetts study). Unless there are also underlying causes, the blues that may color some of the first year or so leading up to menopause are a temporary phenomenon.

Another source of mood changes at this stage is broken sleep. Sweats that awaken a woman several times a night, interrupting REM sleep night after night, can easily produce all the consequences of sleep deprivation. A major function of REM sleep is to allow important brain cells to rest and replenish their chemical stores, according to the latest dream research at Harvard Medical School. It also releases sleep-promoting transmitters and is crucial in regulating body temperature. So it should come as no surprise that a person awakened by temperature aberrations and deprived of the REM sleep needed to reset the body's thermostat is stuck in a vicious circle.

"These are real symptoms. Don't think you're crazy," Dr. Robert Lindsay tells his patients. A good-humored Scottish-born endocrinologist, Lindsay was asked by New York State to set up a bone center in conjunction with Columbia University. His clinic at the Helen Hayes Bone Center is now booked almost a year in advance because, he says, women are not getting reasonable answers to their questions about menopause elsewhere. "The reason estrogen works so well in curing menopausal depression is that it restores REM sleep," he says. "Once women can sleep better, they're fine. They don't need a psychiatrist or a divorce."

To be sure, when Sonja McKinlay went back to do a five-year follow-up of the 2,570 middle-aged women in the Massachusetts study, she had to backtrack somewhat. Women who experienced a long perimenopausal period—more than a two-year transition—had a "moderately increased, but transitory, risk of depression," reports the 1992 paper. And this depression was prompted not by unfortunate social circumstances; it was due to menopausal symptoms. Still, McKinlay holds out against the estrogen deficiency hypothesis. "If estrogen deficiency caused depression, one would expect to see a continued high rate of depression beyond menopause, rather than a transitory peak." But there may be a parallel here between puberty and perimenopause. In both instances the effects on mood can be sharp but short-lived, as the body adjusts to a new hormonal milieu.

There are also life stresses that contribute to depression among women in the menopausal age-group. Chief among those recorded in the Massachusetts study are health problems and high stress. The two groups of women most likely to become depressed are those who have experienced depression prior to menopause and women who have had hysterectomies. "Depression *is* associated with surgical menopause, but it may be the cause rather than the consequence of the surgery since the group of women who undergo hysterectomies is atypical," reports the study. Among those who were found in the follow-up study to have had the highest rates of depression, usually during perimenopause (apart from those with hysterectomies), were widowed, divorced, and separated women with less than twelve years of education. Never-married women showed the lowest rates of depression. Married women fell between the two extremes.

Women who are used to having mood swings with PMS appear to be very sensitive to hormonal fluctuation, Dr. Allen has observed in her practice. "These women may be at risk for depression in the perimenopausal period, when hormonal fluctuations are unpredictable and most violent." Again there is good news: Such women experience great relief when they reach the postmenopausal period. They are released from the treacherous mood baths of their reproductive years and feel a consistency of calmness at last.

The acceleration of bone loss also begins during the perimenopausal phase, as do other changes in the long-term health status of the older woman. "The problem is, nobody *feels* the bone they're losing until it's too late," says Dr. Lindsay. "That is, osteoporosis is without symptoms until it becomes disease."

We build all the bone we are going to make by the time we're thirty-five. "Women really start to lose bone mass at forty," says Richard Bockman, head of the endocrine department and co-director of the Osteoporosis Center at the Hospital for Special Surgery in Manhattan. "And as their hormones fall off, they go through accelerated loss—for about ten years. Then, after the hormones become stabilized, they go back to the normal rate of attrition." Generally, this timetable of bone loss occurs in all white women, according to the Osteoporosis Foundation in Washington, D.C., though not necessarily in women of color.

Similarly, silent changes in the blood vessels that nourish the heart begin taking place during perimenopause. Estrogen makes a woman's blood vessels more elastic. Nature provides this relaxing hormone in abundance during the reproductive years because whenever a woman is pregnant, her blood volume expands. If her blood vessels were as rigid as a man's, the increase in blood pressure would kill both mother and fetus in about the fifth month, according to Dr. Estelle Ramey, professor emeritus and physiologist at Georgetown University.

"So all during your young years, whether you get pregnant or not, you walk around with more elastic blood vessels—until menopause," says Dr. Ramey. When a woman stops producing estrogen, her "good" cholesterol (HDL) level falls. "Bad" (LDL) cholesterol levels start increasing during the transition *into* menopause, as confirmed by the National Institutes of Health. Thus begins for women the narrowing of arteries that will gradually expose them to the cardiovascular disease from which estrogen protected them during their fertile years.

In addition to noticing a lessening of lubrication in the vagina, many women experience bladder problems or suffer the embarrassment of feeling a sudden urge to urinate before they can make it to the bathroom. This "urge incontinence" is common, though little discussed, and may be associated with lack of estrogen. Male urologists usually shun female patients with such chronic complaints. There may be no more than fifty female urologists in the United States. One of them, Dr. Suzanne Frye in Manhattan, says there is a pill called Ditropan that can correct this bladder instability and change a menopausal woman's life.

"But I have cystic breasts, so I can't take hormones, right?" women often asked in our group interviews. Cystic breasts are not uncommon at this stage. Dr. Hiram Cody, one of the top breast surgeons at New York Hospital, explains, "During the perimenopausal period breasts can become lumpier and more tender than before, due to surges of excess estrogen. It subsides within a year after periods stop."

Should women who are suffering the worst symptoms of menopause and accelerated health deficits be able to start hormone replacement therapy during perimenopause? The old dogma says no.

"We know now that there are good medical reasons for some women to begin hormone replacement therapy during the perimenopause years" is how Dr. Allen summarizes current practice. "Acceleration of bone loss begins, risks for coronary artery disease start to increase, atrophy of breast and genital tissue starts. And so most doctors now believe that a woman who is bothered by menopausal symptoms, if she chooses HRT, should be treated before the cessation of her periods."

"STRESS
MENOPAUSE"

It used to be that a reliable guide to when you might expect menopause is when your mother experienced it. But the mothers of today's groundbreaking women knew nothing like the level of workplace stress and environmental toxins we live with today. Acute or prolonged and severe stress can reduce ovarian function and precipitate a temporary menopause at any time from the late thirties on. It may happen around the time of death of a close relative or other traumatic events. The phenomenon is similar to that experienced by a college student up against exams who misses a period.

An anesthesiologist who deals with life and death every day, running an intensive care unit in a midwestern hospital, had her own life turned upside down in her fortieth year.

"I had a fire in my home that was rather devastating," she recounts. Having outstripped her own expectations, she was habituated to a high-performance life. "Of course, I said, oh, well, it was just a fire. I lived in a hotel for six months with two children to care for and continued working very hard—there was my team to run at the hospital—and I was determined that the fire would not have any impact on my life. It was just 'pedal to the metal' and go right on."

Noticing she was a little frantic, the anesthesiologist began vigorously exercising an hour or two daily, in addition to her work and parenting responsibilities. She dropped down to a scrawny 105 pounds and couldn't sleep. "I was anxious and depressed, though I didn't acknowledge it. Suddenly my periods, which have never been that regular, weren't around at all. And when I did sleep, I was waking up five or six times a night and throwing the covers off." Her dentist husband said to her after a few weeks, "Well, honey, I think you're in menopause."

"What! I am only forty years old, of course I am not in menopause." But the very next day she did her blood test. "My FSH and LH were off the wall, and my estrogen was very low," she was chagrined to discover. FSH, the follicle-stimulating hormone, and LH, lutenizing hormone, are responsible for ovulation and under the control of the hormones estrogen and progesterone; elevation of FSH and LH in the presence of low estrogen is indicative of menopause. "It took me about five minutes to put an Estraderm patch on my behind [a means of delivering estrogen through the skin], and within three days I felt my old self again," continued the anesthesiologist. After a couple of months she stopped the exogenous estrogen, and her hormone levels remained normal. "It seems I had a case of temporary menopause, due to much stress," the physician diagnosed herself after the fact. It might also have been precipitated by the extreme weight loss, as found in young marathon runners with low body fat. "In any case," she says, "I look upon that little visit of menopause as one of the greatest gifts that God has ever given me because it made me quite sympathetic to older women."

Everyone wants to be the person she was before. But your body is signaling that this is truly a change of life: You cannot put the same demands on it and expect it to be there for you whenever you have a period of high demand or unexpected stress. You cannot continue indefinitely being the same person as your younger self. To attempt it is the best way to precipitate depression.

Chemotherapy can also bring on a premature menopause. A head nurse at a major metropolitan hospital told me her personal story, which, sadly, is no longer unusual. "I was diagnosed with breast cancer when I was thirty-seven, and I had a mastectomy and a year of chemotherapy. It was the chemotherapy—the drug Cytoxan—that caused ovarian failure."

The most unsettling aspect of this crisis period in the nurse's life was caused by her own—and her doctors'—ignorance about the impact of premature menopause. Known for her natural organizational skills and unflappable temperament, she had organized patient care in a high-demand environment for fifteen years. The untimely menopause caused her months of interrupted sleep and insomnia, along with mounting anxiety and feelings of depression.

"Suddenly, without any change of environment, my organization skills were compromised," noticed the nurse. "I was much slower. It was very troublesome." Once the reason became clear, medication corrected the problems. Some women are lucky, however. Once the chemotherapy is over they do resume cycling naturally. But not all doctors are aware of these complications.

MENOPAUSE MOMS

Boomers having babies in their forties know they have departed from life cycle norms when they have to put on reading glasses to breast-feed. "I can't get him on the nipple without them!" squeals Jane, a former sixties radical turned doting first-time mother at forty-two.

"I am the only self-avowed menopausal mother in my son's preschool" was the amusing confession of Marcia Wallace, an actress who has worked on *The Bob Newhart Show* and *The Simpsons*. Marcia has cultivated the zany image of her celebrity with a red corkscrew-curled mop and loud colors and chandelier-sized earrings. But what struck me were the consequences of reversed life stages that her story represents. A late bloomer, Marcia devoted her young years to pursuing her career and postponed the personal commitments usually made by a woman in her twenties until she reached her forties. She married for the first time at forty-three.

"I figured, by then, all I had left was one egg on a walker," Marcia quips. So she became an adoptive mother two years later. And a mere year after that—guess what? Marcia's new variant on women's life stages might be called the Compressed Life: marriage at forty-three, motherhood at forty-five, and menopause at forty-six.

SEX AND THE

CHANGE - OF - LIFE LOVER

The subject women are least likely to bring up with their gynecologists is any change in sexual interest. The raging hormones of adolescence suddenly become the *un*raging hormones of menopause.

A high-profile movie executive I know went through a major career move in her late forties, the sort of jump that inevitably kicks up gossip: *Was she fired?* One of her best friends warned her: "You know, this could be a very bad mark on your career because people will say, 'She's probably postmenopausal.' You lose your value."

"What are you saying!" The executive gasped in disbelief. "A dried-up, over-the-hill, nasty old me? Do you really think that could be the perception out there?" From a distance, clad in a T-shirt, jeans, and Top-Siders, the slim blond woman could still be mistaken for fourteen.

"Well, you *are* getting older," warned the friend, probably projecting her own menopausal malaise.

"I was flushed with rage," admits the executive. "Because that meant I might be perceived as having no power." She began brooding on her mother's experience. From family pictures she remembered that her mother had been "cute" in her early fifties, but later in that decade, all at once, "her whole face died." So the executive had been spending more time on maintenance: getting her hair highlighted more frequently, going for collagen shots, doing a lot of "teeth things," dropping weight at a ritzy spa. Her first line of defense, she decided, would be to maintain her sex appeal and sexual energy.

"What's amazing is that at age fifty I'm having the best sex I've ever had," she told me confidently. Following a recent divorce, "that part of me has suddenly come to life." What does this have to do with menopause? Everything. Here is a woman who associates sexual potency with power, just like the men who have been her mentors and models at the top of corporate life.

"I made up my mind I'm not going to lose this part," she said fervently. Menopause *will* be held at bay as long as she can keep up her sexual élan.

"Most women after the menopause, if they're reasonably healthy and happy, do not experience a diminution in sex drive," says Dr. Ramey, the senior physiologist at Georgetown University. "But a very large number do—maybe thirty percent," she estimates, adding that the figures are unreliable because doctors don't ask women about their sex drive. "But since we're all living longer, this large number of women who face a diminished sex drive can be a very serious matter."

It is particularly startling for women who have always been sensual to find even slight changes in intimate pleasures they have taken for granted. Gayle Sand is a case in point. A slinky, sexy-looking California woman with great black Diana Ross hair, she flew all the way to Manhattan to have her bone density measured at the Osteoporosis Center at the Hospital for Special Surgery—that's how jittery she was about this thing called menopause.

"I've always been a person that's looked much younger than I actually was. Even now I don't think I look forty-nine years old, do I?" She leaned back in the mean metal institutional chair, attempting a seductive nonchalance, and let the strap of her laminated white tank top drop off one deeply tanned shoulder at the two o'clock point, precisely where the swell of breast tissue started to come up off her ribs. Not an ounce of fat was discernible on her body, nor was there a line apparent in her face. But inside, she was miserable.

"I've always taken really good care of myself. . . . Look, it's like baby skin," she said, holding out an arm glistening like a peeled peach. She was proud of having a DNA glow—all from a diet of boneless, skinless sardines she read about in the seventies in *Cosmopolitan.*

So what was she doing in an osteoporosis clinic, with all those brittle women suffering from low bone mass who have smoked and been slothful about exercise? Well, Sand's own mother had broken her pelvis. But we're not going to be like our mothers, are we? Sand belongs to the first generation of the new fifties woman. She has exercised almost every day of her life. "So I figured I'd postpone all of this. It wouldn't even get to me. The first time I even thought about it was in an exercise class at Sportsclub-L.A. Dyan Cannon, Teri Garr, Magic Johnson, they all go there—it's the stars' gym. I see the tushies of everyone. There's hardly a woman there who has her own breasts. And you can be sure none of *them* ever had *menopause.*"

She was near the end of class, on the floor, grinding the old lower abs into the ground with leg lifts, when she started to perspire profusely. She thought, *What a great teacher!* "But later in the afternoon I was in Gelsons— it's like one of the best supermarkets in L.A.—and I started to have that feeling again. Oh-oh, maybe it wasn't just the great instructor." Dorian Gray time! *You're going to catch me being old.*

Sand was a dental hygienist: "I cleaned the teeth of the stars." She also had a new man in her life, a husband-to-be. She was in her psychiatrist's office when another hot flash hit, so she asked him about it. "If I were you," he said, "I would never mention menopause to this man." She followed the therapist's advice and hid her little secret from the man she married, which wasn't easy once she started having the night sweats.

Just beyond REM sleep—*bolt!*—she'd pop up like burnt toast. A minute later the sweating would start from every pore. Swiftly and silently she'd slip out from under the sheets and take a cold sponge bath, but sometimes her husband would awake and grumble, "Hey, it's wet in here! Jesuschrise, whatsammatta with these *sheets*?"

"I'm just having a little anxiety," she'd say, rubbing his head.

"But then around the same time your vagina starts to get dry. Also, I felt no desire." Now she was talking about a flagging of libido as the estrogen level drops and the tissues of the vaginal wall become thinner and drier. Imagine discussing *that* with your mate, said Sand. "Unless you have a really decent guy, talking to him about menopause is like taking hemlock."

She had learned from reading *Lear's* that yoga was the basis of Raquel Welch's regimen for reaching "balance, calmness, and energy." Of course, Raquel Welch, who at fiftysomething looks like a low-fat-yogurt Lachaise, never mentions menopause. But Raquel does say the secret of remaining a sex symbol forever is yoga. "Change excites me. I am fifty years old. It's when the mind catches up with the body." Along with a diet of Évian water, oat bran, and protein-packed steamed salmon—that's all there is to it!

So Sand slid into bed as if she still belonged to a world of perfectly matched D-cup mango breasts and record arousal times, convinced that all she needed to do to enter the state of fifty-year-old erotica—the state of Raquel-mindedness—was "the mere act of holding a position for a count of thirty or forty seconds." She was thinking, *I'll be a menopause centerfold. I have this glistening body, right?* At the peak of a hot flash—*you want a hot woman? This is a hot woman.* Her new husband maneuvered her into position. And then, *it hurt.*

"It's hard to decide which came first, not wanting to have sex or not wanting it because it hurt," said Sand.

Finally she sat her husband down and told him the facts of life. "I'm going through my Change of Life." Blank look. "I'm going through menopause." Her husband gave her a new name: My Change-of-Life Beauty Queen. She winced; it was a kiss with a kick.

"We find there's a definite major change in sexual response from premenopause to perimenopause," concludes Professor Phyllis Mansfield from her past studies. "The lessening of sexual desire is related to vaginal dryness, which suggests both hormonal and psychological factors."

"Hormones primarily regulate sexual desire in human females," points out Dr. Kim Wallen, the primates researcher at Emory University. "Among monkeys, what we could call middle-aged females are the most socially savvy and attractive to males, and sex is primarily initiated by the female." When the researcher removed half of the estrogen they produce, some of the female monkeys continued to be sexually active, but when he removed all the estrogen, they lost any interest in sex.

Virtually the same phenomenon has been demonstrated at McGill University in studies of women ages thirty to fifty whose ovaries had been surgically removed. Whether or not they took estrogen orally after surgery, they were less interested, less aroused, and had fewer fantasies about sex. But while clinicians collect plenty of data on the frequency of intercourse, they seldom look at the key variable for females: sexual desire.

"There is an overall tendency among doctors to discount women's emotional needs," observes Dr. Wallen. "They will spend a lot of time seeing if there's vaginal atrophy, but they won't spend any time asking about sexual interest or enjoyment." This issue is still not seen as an appropriate part of a menopause workup. Yet a single woman without a regular sexual partner faces a particular dilemma in menopause, since she must be motivated if she wants to find a mate.

The lack of interest in sex may also be due to a decrease in testosterone, the male sex hormone that women's bodies produce in very small quantities. Beyond the fourth or fifth year after menopause, testosterone levels decrease in some women, according to Dr. Barbara Sherwin, associate professor of psychology in the Ob-Gyn Department of McGill University and co-director of the university's clinic in Montreal, Canada. Dr. Sherwin has been conducting research on estrogen-testosterone combinations for fifteen years.

She contends from her studies that testosterone is the hormone primarily responsible for sexual motivation in women, just as it is in men. Very often women will come into her clinic and say, "The kids are gone, my husband and I like each other, we do lots more things together now. But I find I'm simply not interested in sex. Maybe I don't really love him."

These women notice the falloff in desire quite suddenly, says Dr. Sherwin. "When I can date it to the onset of menopause or several years thereafter, or to surgical menopause in women who didn't have that complaint before, we suspect what they are missing is testosterone." The ovary makes one third of the testosterone circulating in a woman's body. The adrenals make the rest, mostly in fat tissue. "So if the woman is thin, she also has less testosterone," notes Dr. Sherwin.

She estimates that in about 50 percent of women, the ovaries stop producing testosterone around the time of menopause. In another 50 percent they go on functioning, and in some proportion of women the ovaries go on overtime—producing more testosterone even than during their reproductive life. These are the women who notice some hair appearing on their upper lips or chins. A woman who wonders about her testosterone level can have it measured from a blood sample; good norms exist.

"Do I have to accept this?" is a question increasingly being asked by dynamic women in their fifties who are at the peak of their careers but alarmed to find their sexual pilot light abruptly lowered. Treatment with very small amounts of testosterone—always combined with estrogen—is beginning to be popular. Dr. Sherwin has had women on this combination of drugs, by injection, for up to twenty years, with good results. She cautions, however, that with a full dose of testosterone about 20 percent developed some facial hair. When she cut the dose in half, to 75 mg of testosterone once a month, less than 5 percent of women had any side effects. When given by injection, testosterone had no effect on HDL and LDL cholesterol levels.

"For those postmenopausal women who find themselves having difficulty with arousal and reaching orgasm, a small amount of testosterone can make a big difference," confirms Dr. Ramey.

When I checked back with Gayle Sand, she had been told by a female doctor about topical estrogen, a very low dose of Premarin used vaginally as a medication to maintain lubrication and keep tissue from thinning in the vaginal walls. "The effects were great," she exclaimed. "I have a normal sex life again." But she had also started a campaign to end the taboo. She'll speak up in an elevator: "Is it warm in here, or am I having a hot flash?" When the occupants gasp, giggle, then cluck, "*You,* you're too young for that," Sand sings back, "No, I'm not. I'm menopausal."

"By and large, the women who have a problem with sexuality in middle life are old married women, like me," believes Janine O'Leary Cobb, editor of *A Friend Indeed,* the Canadian menopause newsletter. (Address: P.O. Box 1710, Champlain, NY 12919-1710.) "Many of us feel we had great sex when we were younger, and we don't mind if we have less now." But Cobb gets letters from women fifty and fifty-two who have taken new, younger lovers. "They're hot to trot and having a lovely time; sex was never so good."

Thus is born a new Old Wives' Tale, in which women pass the word about the tonic effect of a Change-of-Life Lover. The head of a department at a prestigious university was in her mid-forties when she first heard about it from a woman in her mid-fifties. The older woman told her to look forward to menopause: Pregnancy worries went out the window, and she'd had an affair of *grande passion* at that time—starting at forty-nine.

"I was stunned," recalls the younger woman. She was petite and had always prided herself on being taken for younger than she was, but the habit of marriage to a man she had known for several decades had made a buried treasure of her erotic self. Then, suddenly, she found herself swept up in an affair. When? She smacks her forehead with the insight: "It's only now I recognize *I* was the same age! Maybe I thought, *Forty-nine—last chance.*"

Gloria Steinem, known not only as the inspiration of the feminist movement but also as one of the most sexually animated women of her time, was delightfully frank when I asked her what a fulfilling sex life means to her now, having passed fifty.

"I am about to say a series of things that if I had heard them ten years ago, I wouldn't have believed them." She laughed. "All the readers of this should brace themselves—just have faith that it may be true for them, too." She laughed again. "Sex and sensuality—going to bed for two entire days and sending out for Chinese food— was such an important part of my life, and it just isn't anymore. It's still there, but it's less important. I don't know how much of it is hormonal and how much is outgrowing it."

Her still-unlined face seemed more relaxed. She lay back against her sofa cushions, this peripatetic woman who never in the last eighteen years spent more than a few days at a time in her own apartment, and she looked, at last, at home. "It doesn't really matter whether sex goes or doesn't go," she summed up. "What matters is that the older woman can choose whether it goes or not."

EDUCATING

YOUR MAN

Most men go all twitchy when mention is made of anything connected with female reproductive organs. They don't want to hear about your visit to the gynecologist, and they'll do *anything* to get out of making a run to the 7-Eleven to pick up tampons. There seems to be a hangover from primitive thinking that presupposes a woman is unclean when she is in cycle. And if she has "female troubles," the last person she can count on for a supportive ear may be her man. Those deep inner spaces are supposed to be only for pleasuring; they are not meant to have clinical names or flesh-and-blood malfunctions.

In fact, married men are more apprehensive about the effects of menopause on their life satisfaction than women themselves. In a 1991 Gallup poll commissioned by Ciba-Geigy, makers of the Estraderm patch, one in four of the seven hundred women ages forty to sixty expressed concern about menopause, but two thirds of the middle-aged husbands were bothered about it. Only a third of the women were satisfied with their husband's knowledge about the Change of Life, and with good reason. Two thirds of the husbands of premenopausal women expressed fears that their sex lives would be compromised by having a wife in menopause. A majority of the men married to women in the transition focused on the emotional impact on their wives, saying they manifested anxiety, irritability, and mood swings. Fewer than half the men took any notice of physical problems that underlay these emotional reactions, despite the fact that the overwhelming majority of the women in menopause reported struggling with hot flashes, night sweats, and difficulty sleeping.

A gynecological nurse at New York Hospital is struck by how men shun their wives when they come into the hospital for hysterectomies. "The absence of the husband when it's an issue of female sex organs is so common," says Tanya Resilard. "And if they do come to visit, they seem afraid to go to the bedside. They want to be totally separate."

"My husband was incredibly supportive when I had breast cancer, but he really doesn't want to acknowledge I'm in menopause," I was told by a gutsy entertainer. Her spouse is a few years younger than she. When she tries to talk to him about having problems with concentration, he ascribes it to something else—it's stress or money problems or maybe flu—anything but the Change of Life. "He is in major denial about it—why?"

If you are getting older, so is your man. You may represent the mirror of his own aging. Breast cancer a husband can't catch. But aging is sex-neutral. Another woman who felt constrained about admitting to her husband she was struggling with menopause finally realized why. She was the second wife and represented to the husband his own renaissance. "He once told me, 'I don't ever want to think of you as middle-aged.' "

"In certain parts of the South they make you feel really shameful," notes Effie Graham, who grew up in Blanch, North Carolina, and is now a nurse's aide at New York Hospital. "The men refuse to let you sleep in the same room, tell you you're supposed to go through it alone. They had a lot of religious beliefs about menopause. They always said the Lord would take care of it."

In fact, there is much to recommend a woman nearing the end of her reproductive stage. With the passing of pregnancy fears, her lustier fantasies can be played out with a refreshing lack of inhibitions. Best of all—and she must boast about this—she is soon to be free of the "blue meanies" that come with monthly cycles. The Gallup poll findings support this good news: Living through menopause puts far less strain on marriages than the apprehensions would suggest. A nearly identical majority of the husbands and wives polled—70 percent—acknowledged that, in fact, the women's interest in sex had *not* decreased during or after menopause. And two out of five of the women presently in the transition or just past it say that their relationships with their husbands have improved since menopause, while the majority of women reported the quality of their marriages has remained the same.

If there are physical problems or discomforts, they do need an honest airing. The consequences of not being honest with your man about what's going on can magnify the psychological burden and become devastating.

Two middle-aged men came to hear a talk I gave on menopause at a health resort. I was delighted to see them in the audience but curious as to why they would join a group of fifty women. Each of them came to me in his own time to unburden himself.

"I had no idea what women go through in these years," said the trial lawyer, who later stretched beside me after a hike. "My wife may be silently suffering." He sounded seriously concerned, even abashed. "I'm going to talk to her about menopause as soon as I get home."

Another lawyer caught up with me as we were boarding the plane to New York and seemed to need to talk. "I think men need to be educated about menopause even more than women," he said.

"Your wife is a lucky woman," I quipped. My remark set off a shudder of pain in his face, though he said nothing further. Later, over coffee, he told me that his wife had exhibited many of the symptoms I had described. "The sweating at night, insomnia, problems with concentrating. Her moods were up and down, and then mostly down. I had no idea what it was."

Further conversation revealed that his wife had lost her job as a teacher in the recession. Their son had moved out to his own apartment. And she had brought her mother up from Florida to care more attentively for her, but the frail woman had liver cancer and soon died. All in all, a rather typical portrait of the stresses of social as well as physical changes many women experience during the menopausal years.

"I guess I just didn't stop to think how much these losses meant to her. And on top of it, the drain of menopause," he said, flooded with guilt. I tried to comfort him and suggest new approaches for the future. It was too late. One day, four months before, his wife had driven him to their suburban train station for his commute to the city. She knew he had a late dinner with the senior partner that night. When he came home, he noticed the window of the garage door was milky. He found his wife entombed in the car.

The
Menopause
Gateway

*S*ome women have genetic good fortune. Even after entering menopause, they continue to make enough female hormone precursors in their adrenal glands, and to make enough estrogen from these precursors in their fat deposits, so that they do not experience any symptoms or, at most, only temporary hot flashes. This pause is a marker event in their lives, but it does not take on the physical or psychological freight of a major event.

"They are thrilled not to have to deal with the menstrual cycle anymore, and some of them seem to maintain their bone levels very well," observes Theresa Galsworthy, the nurse-clinician who directs the Osteoporosis Center at the Hospital for Special Surgery in New York. Broad-scale figures on the proportion of women who fall into this fortunate group are probably impossible to come by, but activity at the Osteoporosis Center offers a clue. "During the course of the week about fifteen patients come to me to have their bone density measured because they're fairly newly postmenopausal. Maybe two or three of the fifteen have absolutely no symptoms," says Galsworthy. These women are usually on the older side of the norm when they experience the Change, fifty-one or fifty-two.

Women who deal with menopause by denying it entirely become easy to pick out. They are the ones you see lunching on a lettuce leaf and glass of seltzer, their hair color slightly lurid, their time more and more taken up with becoming skillful makeup artists or searching for the right cosmetic surgeon. The results may be admirable and mask the years, but sooner or later time and nature will catch up with us all.

Strenuous dieting at this age, for instance, is the worst way to preserve one's long-term health and grace. Estrogen is stored in the body's fat cells. Some researchers differentiate between the Thin Woman's Menopause and the Plump Woman's Menopause, the latter usually being far less symptomatic. "In populations where women don't get carried away with wearing a size six dress when they're fifty-five, and they still do regular exercise and they're not smoking, bone fractures are not much of a problem," says Dr. Elizabeth Barrett-Connor, a top epidemiologist at the University of California, San Diego.

At the opposite extreme are women who allow themselves to become "victims" of menopause, using this time of life as an excuse to become inactive, go to fat, beg off sex, and sulk, often leading them to depression and the door of menopause clinics. These are the middle-aged women who perpetuate the stereotype of the menopausal woman as synonymous with "mean old bitch."

The professional women I have studied are accustomed to considerable control over their environment, and they have worked hard to achieve it. They pride themselves on being prepared for just about any crisis. These mid-forties dynamos can fax a dinner menu to a caterer, sell a stock, talk supportively to a spouse over a portable phone without missing a step, and remember to take their aerobics shoes to the office along with their satin sling-backs so they'll be able to exercise before appearing glamorous at an evening benefit—all this on the way to argue a case or perform surgery. But they cannot control when they break out in a hot flash or when they bleed.

The meanest loss of menopause, for them, is the sudden loss of control. Among high-performing professionals, puzzlement often develops into panic followed by outrage. That was the route traveled by Meredith, a mother of two and model business leader in her middle-American community, who had stopped counting birthdays at thirty-eight. That was the year she went into business and consciously knew she looked terrific and felt the same way.

She started having mysterious migraines at forty-two. They grew more frequent. Over the next eight years she traipsed around to one gynecologist after another, all of whom posited psychological causes—i.e., "Type A's are often migrainous." At age fifty Meredith was the one to insist upon a blood test that would measure her hormones. She had zero estrogen and zero progesterone. Now completely frustrated, she saw a TV commercial for a menopause clinic in Cleveland, Ohio. She flew there to have a bone densitometer test, which revealed she had 10 percent less bone mass than the norm for women her age. Not one doctor up to then had mentioned her bones in connection with menopause or brought up the risk of osteoporosis.

"I feel like I dropped a percentage point of bone mass in each one of those doctor's offices," Meredith says ruefully. She also wonders, with good reason, if the migraines were the result of estrogen depletion over the past eight years.

I recognized her immediately when we first met. It was the walk, perhaps. Her long legs took the sidewalk one full paving stone at a time, high heels notwithstanding. She was good-looking, still blond and pink-complexioned, the parentheses at either side of her mouth lending animation to her face. Her friends had described her as "dynamic, tough, successful, and doesn't take no for an answer." Her real estate company will do fifty-five million dollars of business this year, and her mortgage banking company will do eighty million.

"You'd think I could manage my period, right?" Meredith wisecracked. Fifty—the number itself—held no menace for her, she said, although it came out that the year Meredith turned fifty, her mother died of breast cancer. It was her first personal experience with death, immediately followed by the onset of her own menopause. "And something happened to me, I don't know what, I became a little nutsy about flying in an airplane. I began to feel a foreshortening of time." Meredith said she was too busy to figure it out.

"I've been obsessed," she says. "Menopause is the only thing that's made me feel I had an age. Because I can't get rid of it. I hate it, big time."

During a group interview, Meredith held up the computerized cost-benefits chart she had designed to analyze whether or not to take hormone replacement therapy. The impressive-looking graph was all the more infuriating to her because there was no bottom line. "So what do I go for? Cancer, osteoporosis, or heart disease?"

For her, menopause represents her lack of control over mortality. Most of us don't have to face up to mortality until our mothers die. The loss of that unconditional love leaves no cushion between ourselves and the outrages of life, no grip against a suddenly perceived slippage on "the downward path" toward one's own inevitable "dusty death." Control becomes magnified in importance. In reaction, Meredith developed her new phobia about airplanes, where as a passenger she could exercise no control. Still, she had pushed away any conscious recognition of her own aging until the physical insults of menopause finally made it impossible to remain, even in her own mind, thirty-eight.

Now, faced with making a medical decision about her own life that involves the breast cancer issue, while the loss of her mother is not yet mourned, Meredith is in a constant state of conflict. She longs to escape from her own success: "Being a mentor is a burden. I feel like I don't live anything new." She resents her husband's assumption that he will take early retirement. " 'What about me?' I feel like saying. 'When can I retire?' " She is unconsciously afraid that she will follow her mother before she has had time to live fully. All these fears and frustrations have been focused on the secondary issue of menopause. And they come out as anger.

To make matters more frustrating, the cost-benefits analysis on how to treat menopause resists adding up to any clear, rational, risk-free answer. Why? Because we don't have enough data. And because everything has a price. A well-informed, affluent woman like Meredith might well decide, "Well, hell, if I know hormones are going to protect my heart, my mind, and my bones, I guess I can monitor my breasts with mammography and my uterus with ultrasound and see how it goes." Or she may prefer to try to manage the whole process naturally.

PARTNERING YOURSELF
THROUGH
A NATURAL MENOPAUSE

Many women resist medicalizing a natural event such as the Change. Others, like Serafina Corsello, have little choice.

"I had a wonderful defense, called denial," admits Dr. Corsello, an elegant European woman who practices nutritional medicine at the Corsello Center on Manhattan's West Side. She was simply never going to have all those unseemly symptoms other women report, poor things. Blessed with high energy and an insatiable desire for learning beyond dogma, Corsello completed a medical internship and residency in New York. Throughout her thirties she juggled a classical medical practice with being a single mother. But in her early forties she became disenchanted with mainstream medicine. The outcome of her mid-life crisis was a commitment to educate herself in complementary medicine—vitamin therapy and other natural procedures—realizing that it meant she would have to study every day for the rest of her life.

"Will I be able to keep up this level of performance?" she worried as she plunged into self-education, taking on new financial burdens as well as committing to a second marriage. But at fifty she found she still had fantastic energy, having always been able to hit the pillow and sleep within two seconds.

"At fifty-two all of a sudden I'd hit the pillow, and hit the pillow—at two in the morning I'd still be hitting the pillow. This was the first sign; it was devastating."

It took Dr. Corsello no time to get an estrogen patch and congratulate herself on re-regulating her sleep. She was herself again for the next two years. "One day I woke up and felt an ominous mass in my breast." The large cyst made her suddenly aware of the history of cancer in her family. She looked at her lovely little patch and pro-gestin pills and said, *"Adieu, chérie."*

She doctored herself with Chinese herbs, indulged in a massage once a week, and concentrated on creating a new aesthetic in her life. She surrounds herself with classical music; even in her office it is constantly in the background, soothing her. Since she loathes exercise but loves dancing, Dr. Corsello built in her own unique daily stress-reducing activity. She shuts the bedroom door while she watches a tape of the *MacNeil/Lehrer NewsHour* and throws herself into high-paced disco danc-ing alone.

Today age fifty-eight, vivacious and utterly charming, Serafina Corsello has just signed a ten-year lease on her office in Manhattan—a powerful statement of her belief that "I'm not only in my prime now, but I'm on my way up." Like many professional women, she is operating under a different time line from her male peers. Her career development was delayed by single motherhood and slowed slightly by menopause. "I cannot stop at sixty, because I have hardly begun," she says enthusiastically. But there is nothing stopping her now. She works every day, and on weekends she studies and writes. "The constant intellectual stimulation allows my mind and body to remain attuned. I keep on improving," she says.

The greatest reward of fifty-plus years of experience, she finds, is mental efficiency. She can actually sense her right and left brains, working in synchrony. And with this wide spectrum of intellectual capacity, she says, "We can zoom in to get the whole picture." She now expresses her ideas on health care *without fear* of offending the male medical establishment. She no longer labors under the younger woman's apprehensions—"What if I'm not right?" or, "Oh, my God, will they be offended?"

"Do you know how much energy this saves?" she says, twinkling. "I used to go into preambles—'you know' and 'on the other hand'—but I've cut fifty percent of that—it's freedom!" As she says now, "If I'm not right, well, I'm not right. This attitude allows you to shortcut all the tangents you had to go through as a young woman—because no longer being a sexual object, you're no longer trying to *please* anybody. At this point what is important to me is elegance. And elegance has nothing to do with sex." The greatest change she has noticed is the aesthetic confidence she has developed as an older woman.

Dr. Corsello has explored most of the herbal preparations popularly used to ease menopausal symptoms. She finds the most effective to be dong quai, a Chinese herbal remedy. "If I'm under stress, bingo, I take thirty or forty little drops and find miraculous relief." She suggests a woman ask a Chinese herbalist to make up a mixture to suppress hot flashes.

Dong quai, the Chinese herb, contains plant sterols that have estrogen-like effects. Plant estrogens are estimated to be one four-hundredth as strong as the estrogen from pregnant mare's urine found in Premarin. Dong quai is available in health food stores in capsules, liquid, or tiny black beans. Siberian ginseng is possibly helpful in opposing fatigue and depressive symptoms. It, too, is available in health food stores. Vitamin E is commonly used to relieve hot flashes. Primrose oil is a recommendation from Dr. Ronald Hoffman, host of *Health Talk* on WOR Radio in New York. It contains gamma-linolenic acid, which helps mediate hormonal activity. Some women report they obtain relief from hot flashes and sweats through acupuncture.

The best natural defense against osteoporosis is to keep the acidity of your blood in proper balance. If you don't, your body will, by removing calcium from your bones to defend the pH balance in the blood. Blood acidity is caused, first and foremost, by chronic stress. Therefore, it is of the utmost importance for any woman over forty-five faced with high-stress professional or personal demands to commit herself to some restorative relaxation measure. It might be biofeedback, prayer, yoga, or routine meditation. Smoking, alcohol, and coffee also raise acid levels in the blood. Carbonated sodas and beef, both of which have a high phosphorus content, are particularly dangerous for postmenopausal women, advises Dr. Corsello. She suggests a diet that emphasizes vegetables, complex carbohydrates, fiber, fish, and vegetable proteins such as tofu.

No natural remedies can be guaranteed effective, and none, of course, is approved by the FDA. Bear in mind that no pharmaceutical company stands to cash in on herbal remedies, since they are natural and can be sold over the counter. And since drug companies fund much of the medical research, it is not surprising that there is no serious money going into the study of Chinese medicine and its impact on menopause.

The pledge to have a "natural menopause," while politically correct, presents some contradictions. Is it "natural" to live for decades beyond fifty? And to want to feel in our seventies the way we do now? This will be the first generation to get old routinely, and one way or another its women will have to provide some things that mother nature did not. None of the herbal remedies protects against bone loss. Janet Zand, a Chinese medical practitioner in Los Angeles, claims that herbs can diminish atrophy of the vagina. But as estrogen levels decline, the vaginal tissues become thinner and drier. Gradually, over the decade of menopause, the vagina will shrink in both length and width. One female gynecologist drew me a picture of the normal, estrogenized vagina of a woman in her thirties. It looked about five inches long and the width of two middle fingers.

"In many women of sixty who have taken no estrogen, I can hardly insert my pinkie," said the gynecologist. Doctors recommend that older women keep up an active sex life because that will keep the vaginal walls elastic. But the common reason that women don't "use it" and eventually "lose it" is that making love becomes naturally painful when the vagina shrinks in size. Estrogen cream, as explained, and new over-the-counter preparations do counteract the problem.

THE HIDDEN
THIEVES

Active women often take pride in toughing it out: "I was too busy to notice menopause—I just sailed right through it" is their refrain. They may not be fully aware of the hidden thieves of menopause: osteoporosis, cognitive changes, and heart disease. This knowledge must be factored in before any of us can make an intelligent decision about how best to manage our own menopause.

Start up a conversation with any group of women in which the ratio of blond to gray has tipped well over the fifty-fifty standoff, and there will be one woman who proclaims righteously, "Hormones? Not me! I want to stay healthy." Another will insist smugly, "I love my estrogen, I wouldn't give it up for anything!" And another will be totally ambivalent, able to be talked into either decision. Elizabeth Barrett-Connor, the University of California epidemiologist, observes that women break down into these three camps.

Most women have become phobic about breast cancer, with some good reason. Their fear, however, leaves them vulnerable to a greater threat. At each group interview I asked the participants to guess what they were most likely to die from. The answers always startled me. Nine out of ten women will say cancer, most of them specifying breast cancer. A few will throw in the possibilities of airline or auto crashes. Almost no one mentions the number one killer of women over fifty.

Heart disease.

In fact, *a woman's chances of dying from heart disease are more than double that of dying from cancer of any kind.* Even as the rise in breast cancer among American women continues apace—one in *nine* women is now diagnosed, and one in four of those will die from breast cancer within five years—cardiovascular disease quietly kills off one in *two* women over the age of fifty.

THE CHEATING HEART

Although the risk of heart attack does not increase abruptly at the moment a woman reaches natural menopause, the rate of heart disease does rise sharply over the course of the decade after a woman reaches her fifties. A clear picture of the "cumulative, absolute risks" of the major causes of death for white women—between the ages of fifty and ninety-four—were spelled out in an editorial accompanying the Nurses' Health Study. There is a 31 percent absolute risk of dying of heart disease, a 2.8 percent risk of dying of breast cancer, a 2.8 percent risk of a hip fracture, and only a 0.7 percent risk of uterine cancer.

"Then why don't we read about women having heart

attacks the way we do men?" someone will sensibly demand.

Perhaps because doctors pay less attention to women's symptoms of heart disease and treat them less aggressively than they do men. As a result, women often develop more advanced heart disease and are more likely to have fatal heart attacks than men. Two new studies involving tens of thousands of patients have recently shown irrefutable evidence of sex differences in the way heart conditions are treated. The unawareness of the general public simply reflects the prevailing attitude in the medical fraternity that heart disease is a man's disease.

"Women lag behind men in heart disease by about five to seven years," says Dr. Bush. "It really starts hitting women in their late fifties and sixties." By the age of sixty-seven they are just as likely to have a heart attack as men the same age, but women are more likely to die from it.

The most significant predictor of heart disease is the HDL level. "Bad" cholesterol levels normally increase in women for some ten to fifteen years following the cessation of periods. Again, dangerous changes in cholesterol count or blood pressure do not announce themselves with obvious symptoms, not until there is a medical catastrophe. "If your HDL level is low, and your LDL level is relatively higher—even if you're walking around with a total cholesterol count of two hundred—you're going to be in trouble," says Dr. Ramey. Estrogen replacement therapy decreases LDL (bad) cholesterol levels and raises the HDL (good) cholesterol levels, each by about 15 percent.

Estrogen has a direct effect on the wall of the blood vessels. "Cholesterol uptake is the first change that occurs in the creation of the plaque that forms the basis for heart disease," explains Dr. Lindsay. "Estrogen appears to block that effect, resulting in open vessels and good blood flow." That explains why estrogen reduces heart disease.

The Nurses' Health Study, the first prospective study of women's health with a population of tens of thousands of women (almost exclusively white), has found striking results on the heart disease front. After ten years, forty-eight thousand of the subjects, who had no histories of cancer or heart disease when the study began, were evaluated. "Women who were taking estrogen after menopause had just half as many heart attacks and cardiovascular deaths as women who never used estrogen," reported Meir Stampfer, who led the study. An evaluation by Dr. Lee Goldman of Brigham and Women's Hospital in Boston concluded, "The benefits of estrogen outweigh the risks, substantially."

EMBEZZLED BONE

The second major thief of menopause is osteoporosis.

Margie is very good at giving care to everyone else—her laundry-toting postadolescent kids and the battered women she works with at the community center in her college town. Still blond, though aware she is white at the roots, Margie will turn fifty this year. "Oh, shit, my number's up" was her reaction. Her doctor told her ten years ago she was a sitting duck for osteoporosis. Small-boned, she remembers her statuesque mother shrinking about seven inches to a mere five feet tall before she died. "I already know I have bone thinning," she admits.

Typically she resists addressing the issue because that would mean her good-bye to youth. "I'll take hormones when I get there."

"What's *there*?" her girl friend challenged her.

"You know, old."

Old is too old to start protecting bones. By the time anybody can *see* osteoporosis, it's too late to reverse it. As you'll recall, we begin to lose bone after the age of thirty-five; the normal rate of loss is about one percent a year. "When you hit fifty, bone loss accelerates to about a percent and a half each year for about ten years," says epidemiologist Trudy Bush, quoting the studies. "Then it levels off again at one percent a year."

Two factors determine a woman's risk of having significant bone loss during this transition. First, her genetic background, and here nature turns the tables on our Western beauty ideal. "I could look at a woman and bet her risks of osteoporosis—fair-skinned, very thin, a smoker, and an early menopause—and usually she'll be symptomatic," says Dr. Lewis Kuller of the University of Pittsburgh School of Public Health.

The second factor is: How strong are the bones a woman has built at her peak? About one third of American women of all ages are calcium-deficient. "The preoccupation of teenage girls is with thin thighs, not good bone, so they get into the habit of drinking diet soda instead of milk," laments Dr. Barrett-Connor. But generational differences here are striking. The frail women who are now immobilized in nursing homes are a different breed from baby boomers who are out there bouncing from work to gym in their nitrogen-cushioned aerobic shoes, popping calcium and snacking on veggies.

Porous bones, which lead to increased risk of fractures, are a major public health problem. One third to one half of all postmenopausal women—and nearly half of all people over age seventy-five—will be affected by this disease, maintains the National Osteoporosis Foundation. Almost a third of women ages sixty-five and over will suffer spinal fractures. And of those who fall and fracture a hip, one in five will not survive a year (usually because of postsurgical complications).

Not only do women die from the consequences of osteoporosis, but it often leaves older women frail, susceptible to falls and broken bones, as well as to the little tortures of hairline fractures in the bones they use for walking and bending—and this by their sixties. Later, in their seventies, osteoporosis makes it painful merely to sit on hipbones pulverized almost into powder; it keeps many women homebound, later even chairbound, and is one of the primary reasons an independent woman will finally succumb to nursing home admission.

Taking calcium supplements *alone* cannot undo the damage done by the loss of estrogen during the period of accelerated loss. And contrary to conventional wisdom, exercise *by itself* is also ineffective in preventing bone loss. These were the results of a study on prevention of postmenopausal osteoporosis reported in the *New England Journal of Medicine* (October 24, 1991). Two regimens were found to be effective. An exercise program *plus* calcium supplements slowed or stopped bone loss. The best results were obtained when estrogen was combined with exercise: Bone mass was *increased*, and other symptoms—hot flashes and sleeplessness—improved after three months.

Vitamin K has been found to inhibit the precipitous loss of calcium in postmenopausal women by up to 50 percent, in a study from the Netherlands. Dark green leafy vegetables like broccoli and brussels sprouts are sources of Vitamin K.

What kind of exercise works for osteoporosis prevention? The slogging pedaler on a stationary bike is not doing her bones much good, and swimming doesn't help, according to endocrinologist Dr. Richard Bockman, co-director of the Osteoporosis Center at New York's Hospital for Special Surgery. The weight of the body has to be carried by the bones in order to stimulate bone strength. Brisk jogging requires a push-off with fifteen pounds or so of one's body weight. Lifting free weights or working out on weight-bearing machines is excellent for the upper body. Some women have back or knee problems that rule out such strenuous activities. What then? "Everyone can walk briskly," encourages Dr. Bockman. "Or do serious walking on a treadmill at a tilt, which gives you both weight bearing and aerobic benefit." Robert Lindsay's study group at the Helen Hayes Bone Center confirms a measurable prevention of bone loss in postmenopausal women treated with 0.625 mg of Premarin plus Provera, even starting at age sixty. "There is pretty good evidence that giving estrogen will slow any further bone loss at least up until the age of seventy-five," says Dr. Lindsay.

Dr. Stanley Birge at Washington University has introduced a radical notion: "The effect of estrogen on protecting against bone fractures may be due to maintaining

high mental functioning." In the OASIS Fall and Hip
Fracture Study, women over seventy who were on estrogen performed better on tasks measuring mental processing speed than women of the same age and education
who were not on the hormone. Dr. Birge postulates that
estrogen-deprived women over seventy are more likely to
suffer the dreaded hip fracture because when they lose
their balance, they don't respond fast enough to break
their fall. "Whereas women of the same age who had
wrist fractures—evidence they did respond and break
their fall—showed twice the mental processing speed."

Technological advances in machinery now make it possible to measure precisely the weight and strength of a
woman's bones. Most major American cities with a medical center or university have a bone densitometer machine (although many are used only for research).
Whatever regimen of calcium and exercise and/or hormones a woman tries can be evaluated against her own
base line, to show annually how much bone she is maintaining or losing. It's the same principle as having annual
mammograms.

"Physicians have to get used to thinking of bone mass
measurement just as they think about a blood pressure
measurement," urges Dr. Lindsay. Some Blue Cross
health plans will pick up part of the cost of osteoporosis
testing. Medicare does not yet reimburse for bone mass
measurement. With regard to bone disease in older
women, we are exactly where we were with breast cancer
twenty years ago—osteoporosis prevention hasn't yet
been considered worthy—another example of the scandalous politics of women's health.

HAS ANYONE
SEEN MY MEMORY?

At forty you can't read the numbers in the telephone book. At fifty you can't remember them. What's going on?

An even more insidious thief of menopause is being quietly noted both by pure-science researchers and by doctors who increasingly hear complaints like those of the very smart best-selling author in Colorado whom I happened to phone one day. "How are you?" I asked.

"I'm thinking slower—are you? I have tremendous trouble concentrating. I start to write and just wander. Am I getting stupid?"

All writers have days like this. But this woman, just past fifty, was usually so witty about life's pitfalls. "What I feel is panic," she said. "I tape every interview now, because I know I won't remember. And I'm so intent on remembering I become extremely irritable. Because if somebody interrupts me while I'm trying to remember, then I'm frightened of losing it."

She wasn't kidding. "You feel less competitive, just slow off the mark." She added glumly, "I think the bottom line is I'm just plain dimmer."

Wait a minute, hadn't she been all smiles after having had a hysterectomy before menopause really hit? "Oh, sure, I was just so glad to be finished with cysts and fibroids, and I was mad at all these doctors." The surgeon told her they had saved one ovary, and it should produce enough estrogen; she wouldn't need to take hormones. That was three years before.

"You might be suffering from estrogen deprivation," I suggested.

"You mean, I'm not stupid, I just need hormones?"

I told her story to Barbara Sherwin, the McGill professor. After the age of forty-eight, she said, that remaining ovary would be quickly withering away. Moreover, manipulation during surgery to remove the uterus often compromises the blood supply to the ovaries. Professor Sherwin said she would be shocked if the writer's estrogen level weren't in the postmenopausal range. And the impact on mental acuity can be quite noticeable.

"Something has happened to my memory," the working women who walk into McGill University Menopause Clinic will often report. They misplace things. It's harder to remember a new phone number, though they always remember the old ones. "People start getting methodical. They don't just put their glasses down on the kitchen counter; they put them down in a specific spot," notes Professor Sherwin. Though this temporary strain on short-term memory is quantifiable, the women are not seriously impaired in their daily functioning.

The few studies that show estrogen loss has a deleterious effect on mental functioning have been done on surgically menopausal women, where the hormonal drop is sudden and acute. For naturally menopausal women, the effect may be a little fuzzy thinking in the early years of Change of Life. "When I was in my early fifties, it was impossible for me to look up in an index and hold three different page numbers in my head," chuckles Canadian newsletter editor O'Leary Cobb. "I'm fifty-seven now, and it's all come back again. Most of us do recover."

Estrogen does help increase the blood flow to the brain. The absence of estrogen has a powerful effect on synapses at certain sites in the brain, confirms Dr. Bruce McEwen, a neuro-endocrinologist at Rockefeller University. He has observed brain chemistry changes in rats during the equivalent of menopause (after their ovaries were removed). "The number of synaptic connections actually decreases. If you administer estrogens, these synaptic connections are remade within a few days." During the female rat's four-day estrous cycle, which mimics the menstrual cycle, these synapses come and go. As for human females, it has been demonstrated that estrogens do have an effect on mental functioning—not on IQ but in terms of performance—though Dr. McEwen is quick to point out our state of scientific ignorance. "No one has bothered to look at cognitive behavior and the effect of estrogen therapy in a long-term study." He emphasizes that the subjective experience of cloudy thinking at times during menopause can be equated, for instance, to jet lag: "It's mostly transient and certainly reversible."

Sure enough, when my writer friend from Colorado went to a gynecologist for her first pelvic exam in four years, the doctor said, "Your vaginal walls are bone-dry." It was immediately obvious from her age that she needed estrogen. "I feel infinitely better, more alert, more moist, more like my old self," she said. Having overcome her initial resistance to HRT, she now believes she will likely live a longer, healthier life. "You get on a track—with regular reminders to get mammograms and Pap smears. If something does go wrong, you have an early-warning system set up to catch it."

DANGEROUS BREASTS

Only a year ago the number of American women diagnosed with breast cancer was one in ten; now it is one in nine. The breast cancer phobia has overtaken almost all other health issues surrounding menopause for many American women, particularly those who have had a brush with it anywhere in their family. As to why we focus more on women with breast cancer than those with heart disease, Dr. Trudy Bush notes that although two thirds of all breast cancers are postmenopausal, one third do occur in younger women, "so you're thinking of the tragic cases among women forty to fifty-two."

A woman I'll call Sarah was brutally widowed in her prime of a dashing, beloved, prominent husband. She was left with a lovely apartment, and a terrace garden she let go to seed because she couldn't bear for several years to step out on it and be assaulted by painful memories evoked by the sun and beauty. Sarah was a freelance commercial artist, and a very successful one. But in her misery she soon became blocked creatively and desperately lonely.

Then to top it off—hot flashes. Hearing about "vaginal dryness" from her friends, she wondered if she would lose interest in sex before she had it again. The whole terror of being identified as a menopausal woman overtook her. "And I'm single, so it matters."

Off to the plastic surgeon for a full face- and neck-lift. Then to the gynecologist for something to "take away the embarrassment of those drippy hot flashes at dinner parties." She had to keep herself shelf-fresh—not like some postdated yogurt—if she was going to keep hope alive for recovering her creativity and her zest for finding a new partner in life.

"But I have these dangerous breasts," she told me, stroking the unusually large, well-formed bosoms under her T-shirt, as if they had grown alien and were ready at any point to turn on her. "I have a history of breast cancer among the women in my family." So, before giving herself hormones, she consulted two other doctors, one a reproductive oncologist. Both said, "Take the hormones. It's worth the benefit."

"But I admit I did it—do it—with great trepidation. Are you on them? Why? Why don't you get off?" The feverish questioning revealed her frustration and suppressed fears. I talked about my primary concern being prevention of osteoporosis and heart disease—the major dangers for older women. Like a number of my most educated and savvy friends, she didn't know that heart disease was the number one killer.

"I also have osteoporosis in my family," she said miserably. "So what do I do? I've been on for five years. My doctor never mentioned any end point."

Doctors seldom do, I said.

"All I know is that once I started taking hormones, the flashes stopped and I had a feeling of well-being. And I looked okay. All that is important to me because I'm an older single woman. So my philosophy has been, If it's working, don't mess with it. But am I doing something to my body that I'll kick myself for later?"

She had a bone density test a couple years before and was told she was fine; the hormones were working. Now she has a new male partner, and she's brought her terrace garden back to life. It's a place of delight where we sat that June day, surrounded by sprouting shrubs and exquisite coral roses, birdsong, and cool breeze. "It gives me such a lift when I wake up to come out here," Sarah said. She's become a happy, healthy, fully functioning, attractive, and sexual woman again. Hormones appear to be integral to her quality of life in her mid-fifties. What risk is she running by taking HRT?

Dr. Estelle Ramey points out that the risk of getting breast cancer rises steadily with age, after menopause, in *all* women, including those who are not secreting estrogen or taking it in replacement hormones—right up to the age of one hundred. Indeed, the single greatest risk factor is age.

Dr. Hiram Cody, the New York Hospital breast surgeon, stresses: "When you're doing a family history, keep in mind that only a first-degree relative—mother or sister—poses an added risk. If it's a grandmother, aunt, or cousin, it's not nearly the same added risk, if any risk at all." Also, to be relevant, one's mother had to have been under the age of fifty when she developed the breast cancer. "It's a *premenopausal* first-degree relative who contributes a significantly increased risk of breast cancer," affirms the leading researcher on menopause in Britain, Dr. Malcolm Whitehead. "Even with the worst possible family history," adds Dr. Cody, "a woman has no more than a fifty-fifty chance of getting breast cancer."

"What we do know is the one-in-nine figure," says Dr. Allen. Speaking as a responsible gynecologist, she recognizes that in prescribing estrogen to one hundred women, it means that eleven of them will be taking a potential growth stimulus to the breast cancer before it is discovered. "Whether this changes the long-term prognosis is not known."

Studies that attempt to document any causative link between HRT and breast cancer are doomed to be inconclusive because the usual dose of Premarin provides only one quarter of the estrogen that a woman's fertile ovaries would produce. But it can be said that the more cycles a woman has, naturally and synthetically, the more estrogen she has in her system over a lifetime.

The primates researcher Kim Wallen points out that for two thousand years most women cycled only two or three times before becoming pregnant, followed by several years of nursing, which again suppressed their periods; then they cycled again several times before the next pregnancies. Historically, then, a woman in her reproductive years may have had a total of forty or fifty ovarian cycles. The modern woman may have more than three hundred. "So human females today are getting a very different pattern of hormonal stimulation," he concludes. "Then, when they go through menopause, we are hitting them with another period of exposure to hormones that they never would have had in the past."

The most complete review of studies on the estrogen-breast cancer link, recently reported by the Centers for Disease Control, found a direct linear relationship: For up to five years of using menopausal estrogen, no increased risk was found. But a woman who uses estrogen pills for fifteen years has a 30 percent greater risk of developing breast cancer. The biological plausibility that ovarian hormones might increase the risk of breast cancer was established one hundred years ago, points out Dr.

Robert Hoover, a National Cancer Institute epidemiologist. "So new data which shows that women on replacement therapy have an increased risk is exactly what you
would predict."

Another expert emphasizes high-fat diets as the chief
culprit in increasing breast cancer rates among American
women. Dr. Caldwell Esselstyn, Jr., is a maverick surgeon
who campaigns for health care "beyond surgery." As
president of the American Association of Endocrine Surgeons, Dr. Esselstyn starts with the data that show nations
which consume greater amounts of fat per person have
the highest mortality rates of breast cancer. "And we
know that rural Japanese women, who still eat a low-fat
diet of vegetables, rice, and a little fish experience far less
breast cancer than Japanese women who have become
urbanized and now like steak and french fries," he says.
"If the lobules and ducts of the breast are constantly being
overstimulated by a high fat intake, which leads to higher
production of estrogen, it stands to reason they will be
more likely to have cell changes leading to cancer."

Not only does a fatty diet add indirectly to the risk of
breast cancer by increasing the estrogen level, but recently basic scientists have demonstrated in the laboratory that fat also has a direct effect on tumor growth
independent of estrogen. Dr. David Rose at the American
Health Foundation in Valhalla, New York, injected human female breast cancer cells into two groups of mice.
He gave one group a diet of 23 percent corn oil, the same
type of fat found in popular margarines. This high-fat
diet both increased and accelerated the growth and
spread of tumors as compared with the low-fat group.
Rose's results, published in the *Journal of the National*

Cancer Institute (October 1991), provide a compelling argument against high-fat diets to protect a woman from *both* heart disease and breast cancer.

"Nobody is arguing against estrogen supplement for the short term—the first three to five years of perimenopause and menopause," says Dr. Kuller, the public health expert at the University of Pittsburgh. "But for the long term, meaning ten to fifteen years, estrogen is drug therapy and should only be prescribed for women predisposed to osteoporosis or heart disease, or both." Dr. Kathi Hanna, senior analyst for the Office of Technology Assessment, a research arm of Congress that has surveyed existing studies, agrees: "It's alarming that practitioners are talking about using hormone therapy indefinitely."

But here's the rub. The key to hormonal protection against heart disease in older women, according to the Nurses' Health Study, was that the healthy women were taking estrogen *currently*. The risks and benefits of estrogen therapy on eight separate health conditions were toted up in a thorough review by T. M. Mack at the University of Southern California. Stopping treatment with estrogen at the end of five years would produce a moderate reduction in the expected hospitalizations for breast cancer. But it would also virtually eliminate all the benefits of long-term health enhancement—a Hobson's choice!

But at least we have choices.

SHOULD I
OR SHOULDN'T I?

So persuasive is the evidence of the multiple protective benefits of estrogen, many experts are now openly promoting estrogen replacement therapy. I asked the premier researcher in Britain, Dr. Malcolm Whitehead, director of the menopause clinic at Kings College Hospital in London and president of the International Menopause Society, "If it was your wife, what would you tell her about coming to a decision?"

"I don't see it as much of a conundrum, perhaps because I'm a man," he opines. "If estrogens really do reduce coronary-artery-disease death by fifty percent, that factor alone will swamp any other factor in the equation." Dr. Whitehead openly envies women for *having* a choice; men don't. "We are stuck from the time we're born to the time we die with arterial disease as a sword of Damocles hanging over us."

Some top researchers are even reversing themselves on the conventional prescription for *combined* hormone replacement therapy. The progestins continue to present a problem. The best data from the United Kingdom (by Roger King and Tom Anderson at the Imperial Cancer Research Fund) indicate that the effect of progestins on breast tissue either is neutral or may slightly increase the risk of cell division. "One would predict that, because women get lumpy breasts before their period, when progesterone is at a high level in the bloodstream," affirms Dr. Whitehead.

Dr. Robert Lindsay, the osteoporosis expert, is not an enthusiastic supporter of progestins. "If you give ten milligrams of Provera in combination with the Premarin, many women feel premenstrual and crabby and irritable. They call up and say, 'Why did you give me that stuff?' The concern is that many people who would gain in healthy active years, on estrogen replacement, are turned off by the required addition of a progestin and the continuation of periods."

The reason to use the progestins is to protect the uterus. Estrogen used alone has been clearly linked with an increased incidence of uterine cancer. Abnormal bleeding patterns may be able to warn early of precancerous changes in the lining of the uterus. However, this early sign does not always occur, warns Dr. Allen. Fortunately the uterine lining is not difficult to monitor. Endometrial biopsy and/or a D&C are useful and easily performed. Recent findings suggest that ultrasound may be able to monitor the uterus lining as well. There is a high cure rate for uterine cancer that is caught early.

There are now at least a dozen different regimens recommended by doctors for combining estrogen and progestin. No two women respond the same way. "I always tell people the first year is trial and error," says Barbara Sherwin at the McGill University clinic. "We're constantly readjusting the dose, the types of products, and the regimen." Cycling the progestin throughout the month, for instance, allows a woman to use a lower dose, and after six months or so, periods generally cease. "In some women that works very well, but we don't really know yet if it reduces or eliminates the risk of uterine cancer," adds Dr. Lindsay.

A new way of administering the counter-hormone is progesterone in an oral micronized form, which is the only way the body can absorb the *natural* hormone. The progesterone in this product comes from either the South American yam or the soybean plant. "It doesn't have all the negative side effects of Provera but many of the positive effects you're looking for from a progesterone," enthuses Dr. Jamie Grifo, a new-generation gynecologist at New York Hospital. He and Dr. Notelovitz in Gainesville believe oral micronized natural progesterone is the wave of the future. A study on twelve women with moderate to severe menopausal symptoms by Dr. Joel T. Hargrove at Vanderbilt University Medical Center tested the safety of a daily combination of natural oral micronized progesterone (200–300 mg) with estrogen. After six months the combination improved symptoms with minimal side effects and left the women with a thin endometrium and no evidence of suspicious changes in tissue. Also, withdrawal bleeding stopped. It also raised the good cholesterol (thereby eliminating the counterproductive effects of synthetic progestins on the heart disease protection offered by estrogen).

The Women's International Pharmacy in Madison, Wisconsin, is the only U.S. outlet for oral micronized progesterone (OMP), produced by Upjohn. Wally Simons, a pharmacist there, says that synthetic progesterone is from ten to a hundred times as potent as the natural micronized product; therefore, the equivalent of 2.5 mg of Provera is between 25 and 250 mg of oral micronized progesterone.

The British expert Dr. Whitehead is not so optimistic about oral micronized progesterone. "In our experience

OMP causes sleepiness and lassitude when given in dosage high enough to ensure endometrial protection." (In a dose-ranging study he did at Kings College Hospital, 300 mg of OMP a day for ten days was necessary to reproduce the effect of the body's own progesterone during the luteal phase of the menstrual cycle. Although a 200 mg daily dose will suppress cell duplication, it does not produce the full secretory transformation of the uterine lining.)

"What does a woman do, then, if the only dose that protects her makes her fall asleep?" I asked Dr. Whitehead.

"Then you have a problem."

Acknowledging the problem, Meir Stampfer, the principal investigator on the Nurses' Health Study of heart disease, writes, "An important challenge is to develop a progestin regimen or formulation that will maintain protection of the uterus, yet not impair the benefits of estrogen on lipids." The British and Europeans have more progestin agents available than do American physicians. Dr. Whitehead favors a Dutch-made agent, derived from the natural progesterone, called Duphaston, made by Duphar in Holland and licensed for use in the United Kingdom. "It gives you good protection of the uterus, but in our experience, it causes few adverse symptomatic and psychological effects and gives you little of the reduction in cardio-protective effect."

The Estraderm patch is an increasingly popular method of delivering estrogen to the body. A small adhesive bandage releases the hormone through the skin, with the advantage that it maintains a continuous, consistent level of estrogen in the system, like a time-release capsule. It is not metabolized through the liver and therefore has no impact on digestive diseases. The FDA recently approved Estraderm as a treatment for menopause and osteoporosis. Estrogen delivered in this form, however, has not proven to be as beneficial in protecting against heart disease as estrogen taken orally.

American physicians may eventually move away from progestins, suggests Dr. Lindsay. Two other respected American experts agree. "We're hypothesizing that unopposed estrogen is better than an estrogen/progestin regimen," says Dr. Trudy Bush of the Johns Hopkins School of Medicine. Dr. Bush, together with the epidemiologist Elizabeth Barrett-Connor, pushed the U.S. government to fund the first limited study to measure the health risks and benefits of hormone therapy on women in menopause (Progestin-Estrogen Prevention Intervention, or PEPI). The PEPI study will have results in 1993.

Other experts I interviewed were against hormones being given routinely to menopausal women. They remember the alarming rise in uterine cancer in the early 1970s following by several years the celebration of hormone therapy in various women's magazines and in a 1966 book, *Feminine Forever*, whose author's foundation received funding from at least one drug company. Subsequently, uterine cancer has declined.

The debate over "natural" vs. "medicalized" menopause will only grow more vigorous as boomers come along. I was asked to give a talk in San Diego to women state legislators from all over the country on the subject of menopause. It was quite amazing: Four hundred busy political women stayed for several hours on the last Sunday of their conference to discuss every aspect of the Change. Many of them came up to the microphones to describe their experiences. One lawmaker from Minne-

sota told how a group of her peers in the state capital decided they weren't going to skulk around and hide their
postmenopausal status—they were going to flaunt it. So
they formed a bike club and rode to the statehouse wearing Day-Glo pink T-shirts with THE HOT FLASHES printed
in black letters across the front. Finally, Betty Friedan
took her turn and pooh-poohed the whole subject. Hormones were dangerous, and besides, who needs them?
Drawing only on her own experience, she shrugged. "I
may have had a hot flash, one hot flash, while I was giving
a major speech in the middle of the seventies."

But no woman's genetic makeup should be held up as
the model for abstinence from hormones, making the
next woman feel lesser for having a different nervous
system, different metabolism, and different stores of hormones, just as she has different depths of pigment and
strands of DNA in the tangle of her own creation.

"We wear glasses when our eyes are bad, we use hearing aids, we get false teeth, and now we're putting in new
knees and hips," counters Columbia University physiologist Fredi Kronenberg, a researcher in rehabilitation
medicine at Columbia University Hospital of Physicians
and Surgeons. "Estrogen affects our hearts, our minds,
our bones, our behavior, and our sexual function and
desire." Her basic argument is, How can women expect
to live fully for thirty-five more years and *not* supplement
the estrogen they no longer make naturally?

Several studies indicate that women live longer if they
are on estrogen, notably the Leisure World Study of 8,881
women ages 40 through 101 in a Southern California
retirement community. The women completed a health
survey in 1981 and were followed up seven years later.

Twenty percent fewer of the women with a history of using estrogen had died from any cause, compared with those who had never taken estrogen. The more startling evidence, reported in 1991, is that the longer the women used estrogen replacement therapy, the lower was their mortality risk. Current users who had taken estrogen for more than fifteen years enjoyed twice the benefit—a 40 percent reduction in their overall mortality.

"Women with symptoms certainly feel better when they take estrogen, and those in professional positions almost always feel they work and concentrate better," concludes Dr. Lindsay. The standard comment volunteered by British women who have been on long-term hormone replacement therapy, according to Dr. Whitehead, is: "They say they feel fit, and they always seem to have four times as much energy as their neighbors do."

To make it easy for your doctor to take care of you during these years, know what you want. Here are questions to ask yourself:

- Is there any evidence of osteoporosis in your family?
- Did your mother or a sister have breast cancer? How young? Was it estrogen-sensitive?
- Is there any family history of heart disease?
- Is there a family history of cancer of the uterus?
- Did you have serious PMS?
- How long have you been perimenopausal? (The longer it takes you to move from irregular cycles to no cycles, the more likely you are to have physical and emotional symptoms.)

· Rank in order, on a scale of one to ten, what
concerns you most about menopause—i.e.,
No. 1 might be the embarrassment of having
hot flashes in public, and No. 10 might be
the fear of breast cancer or of losing memory
and concentration.

If you have had a pre-cancerous condition in the cervix,
not to worry; cervical cancer is not hormone-dependent.
Also, there is no evidence that estrogen increases the risk
of ovarian cancer.

COST-BENEFITS OF HORMONE REPLACEMENT THERAPY

Risks	*Benefits*
1. Possible increased risk of cancer of uterus	1. Prevents osteoporosis
2. Unknown associations with breast cancer	2. Decreases heart attacks
3. Continued menstruation possible	3. No hot flashes
4. Breast swelling or pain	4. Decreases insomnia
5. Premenstrual-like syndrome on progesterone	5. Improves energy
6. Expense of doctors' visits and tests for screening	6. Improves mood and sense of well-being
	7. Restores sexual interest and comfort
	8. May improve concentration and memory
	9. May improve longevity

D O   I   H A V E

T O   S T A Y   O N

H O R M O N E S   F O R E V E R ?

One of the scare statements often repeated is that hormones will only put off the inevitable. "A woman who starts on hormones will have to stay on forever because if she stops, all the menopausal symptoms will return with a vengeance," a prominent New York gynecologist told a new patient. This "express train" scenario is false, says Dr. Lila A. Wallis, a New York internist with forty years of clinical experience. Many older patients have grown into their sixties under her care as users of hormone replacement therapy.

"In the very early menopause, women require larger doses of estrogens in order to control their symptoms," says Dr. Wallis. "As they get older, the estrogens can be cut down and the patient is more tolerant of the decreased dose."

The one action to avoid is to go off hormones "cold turkey." The operative generalization is this: *The more abrupt the drop in estrogen, the more severe are the symptoms.* This explains the severity of symptoms often reported after a hysterectomy or during a sudden, stress-related menopause, just as it explains the flare-up of symptoms that may occur if a woman who's been suppressing them for a decade with HRT abruptly discontinues the hormone bath to which the body is accustomed. There is a simple way to avoid this problem: tapering off. Dr. Wallis advises her older patients to watch the "pause" at the end of the month and note whether or not hot flashes or any other symptoms resurface. As symptoms subside, the regimen of replacement hormones can be gradually reduced. The body is allowed to adjust over time.

HELP IS
ON THE WAY

The politics of menopause are at last being challenged by female health professionals and lawmakers. Congresswoman Patricia Schroeder and the Congressional Women's Caucus pushed for the first subcommittee hearing on the role of menopause and disease, which took place in April 1991. Under the glare of publicity, the government responded. Dr. Bernadine P. Healy, named director of the NIH a few months earlier, has boldly spearheaded a massive clinical study to close the vast knowledge gaps that surround the health of older women. She readily admitted in 1991, "Even now . . . physicians still do not have enough scientific information to respond to a woman's questions about postmenopausal hormone replacement therapy." Congress has already appropriated twenty-five million dollars for the NIH study. Ten years down the road, Healy promises, we will have more of those answers.

A committee member at the first menopause hearing opined that the Women's Health Initiative would be too late for his wife, who's in her fifties now. "I just hope we have results in time for my daughter."

What can you do?

We can all help to break the conspiracy of silence about menopause by starting self-help groups and sending out educational messages in every way, shape, and form. There is also an opportunity for each state to piggyback its own questions, specific to that region, on the National Institutes of Health questionnaire. The NIH is contacting women's health centers and clinics around the country to set up over fifty study groups. Individuals can assist in recruitment drives for women to be subjects. We will render normalcy to a normal transition only by talking about it and sharing what we do know and what we are determined to find out.

If we approach this journey with optimism, determined to become informed consumers of health information, and choosy about the physician who will work with us as a partner in managing a natural life transition rather than expect a compliant "patient," most of us can live and love and work and cope quite well. Here are three important ways to think about the passage through menopause:

First, consider the time you have left to live—one half your *adult* life. If you have the good fortune to reach menopause, you have a responsibility to educate yourself on how to preserve your physical and mental well-being so that your older years can be vigorous and independent. Think of going for the long ball. Take a life review of where you have been, the parts of yourself you have already lived out, and those yearnings you left behind as a girl. How can you put play back into your life? How can you turn your talents and life skills to caregiving in the broader, even worldly sphere? What adventure of mind or heart or bold personal challenge would your ideal future self dare to take? Consult her; then follow her lead!

Second, find a topnotch physician partner to help you manage your menopausal transition. Most doctors will tell you if you ask them honestly: How many women do you treat over the age of forty-five? (That will tell you how interested or experienced the physician is in treating menopause.) Ask the doctor to describe menopause to you. Then ask questions. If your inquiries are brushed off with pat or curt answers, walk away. There is no clear menopausal test. If you want some hormonal guidelines, the tests to ask for are your estrogen level and LH and FSH levels and an osteoporosis screening. But your best guide is your own symptoms.

Be an inquiring, even challenging partner, not a passive follower of doctor-as-God. Decisions on how to plan for the health and well-being of your next thirty years or more cannot be made in a twenty-minute visit with your doctor, any more than you would decide on the purchase of an expensive car in that time. Expect a year of trial and error.

Third, take charge of the transformation. That means becoming serious about regular exercise. Find something you like to do: best if it requires making an appointment or a social date because then you'll have to keep to it, but you can also park at the end of the mall and walk briskly with march music on your Walkman. This physical effort will support your bones, heart, lungs, as it pumps oxygen for clear thinking and endorphins for good feeling straight to your brain. Transformation also means looking for ways to stop pushing yourself so hard professionally or inviting so much stress. It may help to find a therapist or a group to work with in identifying the woman you want to be for the rest of your life. Finally, this momentous passage invites meditation and spiritual exploration. A wisewoman will make time to contemplate things eternal and appreciate the life she has.

Coalescence

―――――

*O*nce the ovarian transition is complete, a woman enters a new state of equilibrium. Her energy, moods, and overall sense of physical and mental well-being should be restored, but with a difference. Think of it as discarding the shell of the reproductive self—who came into being in adolescence—and coming out the other side to *coalescence.* (*Coalesce* means "to come together," "to unite"; -*escence* denotes "action or process," a change state.)

It is a time when all the wisdom a woman has gathered from fifty years of experience in living comes together. Once she is no longer confined to the culture's definition of woman as a primarily sexual object and breeder, a full unity of her feminine and masculine sides is possible. As she moves beyond gender definition, she gains new license to speak her mind and initiate action.

The time sense changes. People in their late thirties and early forties are commonly pursued by a frantic, hurry-up feeling—as if everything they have missed out on must be seized immediately or lost forever. This midlife agitation is often revived for women by the perimenopausal panic in the mid to late forties. As suggested, the foreshortening of time sense takes place because the forties represent the old age of youth, while the fifties open up the youth of Second Adulthood. What may have been seen as a dead end is now perceptible as a gateway to years ahead that spread out like a brand-new playing field.

"I spent a large part of my early adult life on logistics—just getting from point A to point B with three young children and no money," said an animated fifty-nine-year-old schoolteacher, describing her postmenopausal change of outlook. "Now, with no responsibilities, with three functioning children who are off on their own, it's a liberation that is difficult to explain . . . it's emotional, physical, financial—total."

We have a second chance in postmenopause, unencumbered by the day-to-day caregiving and thousand and one details of feeling that most women pour into the long parental emergency, to focus on the things we most love and to redirect our creativity in the most individual of ways. We must make an alliance with our changing bodies and negotiate with our vanity. No, we are never again going to be that girl of our idealized inner eye. The task now is to find a new future self in whom we can invest our trust and enthusiasm.

Today's "coalescents" are mapping out a whole new

stage of life. Despite all the idiosyncrasies of this age-group, common refrains emerged in the stories given by women in their fifties:

"Making choices is so much easier" was a comment echoed from coast to coast.

"You don't get your period, *and* you don't have to panic when you don't," summed up a West Coast woman.

"You don't have to play the girl game anymore," said an attractive divorcée who's let her hair go gray. "But it's still all right to be a vulnerable female person and allow yourself moments of weakness. Now it's *your* choice."

The "empty nest," which we were told by psychoanalytic theorists would leave us feeling useless and lacking in self-concept, turns out not to register as a main concern in large-scale contemporary studies. When women mentioned it at all in interviews with me, it was usually with relief or relish.

"After being liberated from keeping those five long-legged sons filled up, a new world opened up to me as I approached fifty," said a southern woman who had happily fulfilled the duties of a full-time wife. "One of the kids said, 'Mom, what are you going to do with yourself now that we're all gone?' I said, 'Hon, I don't know, but count on it—I'm going to have fun!' "

"The freedom of middle age is fantastic!" exulted a former homemaker who loves her new life as a real estate maven. "Now *Mom* can lie down before dinner. Or I can pay somebody else to do dinner. Or I don't have to have dinner at all."

"Watch out, I'm heading downhill and I'm on a roll!"

called a Colorado woman as she passed me on the jogging track.

A great discovery of the fifties is the *courage to go against*—against conformist behavior and conventional wisdom. A woman can at last integrate the rebellious boy in herself, left behind back when she was ten or eleven and eager for adventure and before she became vulnerable—i.e., capable of being violated. Social psychologist Bernice Neugarten reports that as women move into later life, they become more accepting of their own aggressive and egocentric impulses and feel less guilty. Research on female cognition has demonstrated that women shift more fluidly than men from intellect to intuition, or from linear to nonlinear thinking, seeing the events of life as less black and white than as a continuum. Given the added status and confidence of the postmenopausal state, women are in an optimal position to voice their convictions and make a powerful public impact. An initial sense of timidity and danger may give way to relief and excitement as the new older women realize there are still many "firsts" ahead. Once they stop clinging to a life and conditions that have been outgrown, they can stake out their freedom at last. This usually happens by the mid-fifties, as is evident in the following excerpts from interviews:

"I'm not pulling my punches like I used to—I'm saying more of the things I really think," boasted a beautiful Rochester woman, now sixty-eight, who has remade herself into an organizational management executive.

"I grew up mechanical—I could fix a flat or repair

the roof, but I always deferred," admitted a well-built African-American woman of sixty who takes care of a three-family house. "Now I don't need anybody to tell me how."

"You have the whole spectrum of intellectual capacity to draw on," enthused a physician who left conventional medicine and is enlivened in her late fifties by practicing nutritional medicine.

Such comments hint at the welcome change of perspective as women come through the disequilibrium of menopause into the stage of mastery that follows it—a passage that is not cause for remorse but for celebration. In fact, my previous studies of life stages on sixty thousand adult Americans established that women in their fifties, by self-report, had a greater sense of well-being than at any previous stage in their lives. A considerable body of psychological study data has accumulated since then, confirming that women are least likely to be clinically depressed in middle age.

EXTRA-SEXUAL
PASSIONS

At a small conference on "The New Older Woman," organized by Group Four, a consulting partnership, and held at the Esalen Institute in summer '91, prominent American women from diverse backgrounds and professions were invited to share viewpoints on what it's like to be energetic, ambitious, optimistic, and over fifty in today's America. Most said they had negotiated the passage through menopause with a minimum of difficulty. The happy little secret they shared was that they had enjoyed the best sex of their lives during and just after menopause, between the ages of forty-five and fifty-five. (Granted, their generation had been sexually repressed in youth.) These were also women of a generation totally unschooled in what to expect of menopause. The usual comment was that they were "too busy" with career, personal relationships, or family to dwell on the physical or psychological accompaniments to the Change of Life.

Participants now in their sixties or older agreed that there came a point, sometime in their fifties, when they had to let go of—or at least had to stop trying to hang on to—their youthful image. Although it was painful at the time, they had all found a source of new vitality and exhilaration—a "kicker." As each one described her personal struggle, a common denominator emerged and the group hit upon something profound:

The source of continuing aliveness was to find your passion and pursue it, with whole heart and single mind. It is essential to *claim the pause* and find this new source of aliveness and meaning that will make the years ahead even more precious than those past.

For several of the women the passion was to correct an ignored community or societal wrong: Harriet Woods, for example, the former lieutenant governor of Missouri, had lost a Senate race and turned to creating a brand-new political institution, a think tank at the University of Missouri. She went on to become president of the National Women's Political Caucus, the only bipartisan national membership organization that recruits, trains, and supports women for elective and appointive office. In both roles she pursues her passion: to help women learn to use power in ways different from hierarchical, victimizing male models, with an eye to transforming society. "Age no longer has the same relevance it used to have," she affirms. "Whether it is through caregiving or creating new institutions as I just did . . . it happens for women who are beyond what was once thought of as the curve for making a contribution."

Others had found more private passions: going back to school to finish a degree, writing a book, or the pursuit of knowledge in a special field for the pure pleasure of knowing.

It was agreed that the older woman with fewer resources often feels isolated, even cheated. Just as she feels free to pursue personal goals, her husband may be going into decline or physical dependency; returning children may try to manipulate her into remaining chief cook and laundrywoman; divorce or ailing parents may cramp her financially. But although these realities might sound like arguments against risk-taking at this time of life, in fact, they make it all the more essential to dare new explorations.

Vi Beaudry defied all these assumptions about the "trapped" menopausal woman, who is expected to feel too little self-worth to dare a divorce at such a precarious stage. Rather, her life started again in postmenopause, and it wasn't because she had an easy passage or plenty of money or fancy degrees. We met in a blue-collar redneck section of a southern city, the sort of place where Vi might stop for a light driving down Dixie Highway and suddenly have a hooded Klansman in her face, thrusting literature through her window. When it happened, this steel magnolia pressed her gator boots to the gas pedal and just drove on. There is very little that makes her afraid anymore.

"It was my *husband* who had himself a menopause, okay?" she explains. Some pause. He sat down in front of the TV and didn't get up for the next ten years. And it wasn't paid retirement. Vi was in her late forties when the siege began. She was the one having night sweats, but there was no time to indulge herself. Having done volunteer and unpaid political work while her children were still at home, Vi, as an overweight high school graduate, had to retool herself to enter the job market in a hurry. She tinted her hair strawberry blond, sewed herself a flattering wardrobe, and eventually moved out of clerking by creating a job for herself with the local cable company as its community services director.

"This time of menopause, just when you're expected to be falling down, you have to become self-supportive enough—economically, emotionally, spiritually—to go out on your own, if you have to, and start another life," she has learned. On her fifty-seventh birthday, possessed of the postmenopausal courage to confront, Vi shook her husband out of his long day's TV doze.

"Today is my birthday," she announced. "My mother died when she was five years older than I am now. I do not want to live the rest of my life like this."

"What does your birthday have to do with it?" he said.

Okay, he didn't get it. She went into the kitchen and set down the clipboard that attested to her new authority as a member of the district sewer board. She looked at the rings flashing on her fingers and felt the gold lanyard looped around her semi-sheer blouse; she had bought them herself, all of it. It was quite a revelation: She did not need a man to live, and she wasn't living with a man. Vi went back and gave her husband an ultimatum. "I would like for you to contribute something to the running of the household by September first." When the date came and he demurred, Vi filed for divorce.

"I had a lot of readjustment to do," she admits. She had just paid off the mortgage on the house, but community property divorce laws forced her to mortgage it again. Vi needed a couple of years to rise above her anger. "But rather than be bitter about it, hey, you're buying back a life—not just holding on to a mortgage that would make you a prisoner for the rest of your life."

Neighbor women, still very southern in their ways, keep waiting for Vi to become depressed, feel socially invisible, go to seed. She laughs. "There are a lot of things worse than going home to an empty house." Hardly invisible, now sixty, she runs the community arts festival, sits on several community boards, and is one of the most lusty, healthy, outspoken, self-confident people in town.

How—or if—one *welcomes* postmenopause, and consciously prepares for the new freedom it offers, makes all the difference in reaping the benefits of the stages beyond. The gateway to our Second Adulthood is a passage to be approached with pleasurable anticipation, as we take control over our lives and assume the new license to be outrageous. Anthropologist Mary Catherine Bateson counsels: "Say to yourself, I'm going to start a new life. It could be a stage of expansiveness or withdrawal. It could be a time of introversion or of worldly adventure."

WISEWOMAN POWER

Women who no longer belong to somebody now can
belong to everybody—the community, a chosen circle of
friends, a worship group, or even the world—by virtue of
contributing knowledge or creative insight or healing
gifts. In fact, the elder women who survived in ancient
or tribal cultures developed a way to further species survival *independent* of their wombs. These women became
sources of experience and wisdom and were often venerated as shamans with healing powers, upon whom both
individuals and tribe depended to handle crises. As the
influence of female deities increased steadily up to about
500 B.C., the role of medicine man was assumed by medicine woman. "The fact that women were shamans during
this period indicates they had entered into the most au-
thoritative and honored ranks of healers," writes Jeanne
Achterberg in *Woman as Healer.*

Wisdom, or the collective practical knowledge of the
culture that is more simply termed common sense, has
continued up through history to be associated with older
women. Even in premodern times, when Christianity re-
jected females as deities or primary healers, great public
women did emerge and exert their influence through the
religious system. Some became prized as advisers to em-
perors and popes, turned to for their healing powers,
venerated as holy—and it turns out that they were usually
near fifty when they took on this aura of wisewomen.

Today's pioneering women in postmenopause in advanced societies eventually give up the futile gallantry of

trying to remain the same younger self. Coming through the passage of menopause, they reach a new plateau of contentment and self-acceptance, along with a broader view of the world that not only enriches one's individual personality but gives one a new perspective on life and humankind. Such women—there are more and more of them today—find a potent new burst of energy by their mid-fifties.

Margaret Mead spoke frequently about postmeno-pausal zest and regarded it as a widespread phenomenon. When Mary Catherine Bateson was writing her own book *Composing a Life,* she was unable to find a formal discussion of the phenomenon mentioned by her mother. Yet Dr. Mead certainly experienced a grand bloom in her fifties, following on a shattering series of blows in her forties.

When the bomb exploded over Hiroshima, Mead tore up every page of a book she had nearly finished. As she wrote in her autobiography, *Blackberry Winter,* "Every sentence was out of date. We had entered a new age. My years as a collaborating wife . . . also came to an end." She was forty-three. Her adored husband left the marriage, her closest colleague died, and she spent several years devising a new way of working without them, while improvising a life as a divorced professional mother of a small child.

But between the ages of forty-five and fifty-five, as Bateson pieces together the famous anthropologist's history, "she seemed to become prettier, she bought a couple of designer dresses for the first time, from Fabiani, and I think she started a new romantic relationship. Without question, she went through a complete professional renaissance." Boldly Dr. Mead decided to return to the field at the age of fifty-one. She boned up on languages she had learned twenty years before and went back to New Guinea, forging a major intellectual new start with groundbreaking research on social change published in the book *New Lives for Old.*

In fact, hormonal changes may partly explain why so many women describe a vastly increased store of energy after menopause, while some men move toward despair and decline. A good deal of the energy of a younger woman goes into producing enough of the hormone progesterone to sustain a possible pregnancy. Postmenopausal women no longer suffer from the handicap of continually fluctuating levels of progesterone. Menopause also puts an end to the mood swings of the menstrual years.

Middle-aged men have no such abrupt shutdown of hormone production and no accompanying surge of energy. "In my view, it's not so much that men decline as that women start to overtake them," posits Dr. Katharina Dalton, a leading British endocrinologist. "It is also a medical fact that men's bodies age far faster than women's. . . . Middle-aged men do not experience the new lease on life, the sense of liberation that postmenopausal women often enjoy. Their health gets worse, while that of their wives gets better."

This fact places many middle-aged wives in the role of woman-as-healer. They don't need the status of a prehistoric medicine woman or that of a medieval abbess to tap into their postmenopausal powers of active imagination, whereby they may be able to lead a seriously ill spouse or parent toward self-healing or spiritual comfort.

There is even a hormonal explanation to underscore the observation across cultures of the switch in male-female behavior during middle age, a phenomenon I've called the "Sexual Diamond." From their mid-forties to their sixties, women tend to become more aggressive and goal-oriented, while men show a tender and vulnerable side that may have been formerly suppressed. Women whose ovaries have stopped putting out the female sex hormone estrogen still produce in the cortex of their ovaries a small but consistent amount of the male sex hormone, testosterone. The relatively high level of testosterone in about 50 percent of postmenopausal females could partially explain the take-charge behavior so often exhibited by middle-aged women. Meanwhile, men's testosterone levels are gradually decreasing with age.

"Do you know how you feel a week after your period ends—like you could climb mountains and slay dragons? That's how a postmenopausal woman feels all the time, if she's conscious of it," says Elizabeth Stevenson, a Jungian analyst in Cambridge.

Stevenson had a year of hot flashes, which she relieved with acupuncture, and by the age of fifty-two broke through to a state of postmenopausal zest. "It's both physical and psychological," she says. Now fifty-five, she doesn't have the same energy level she had at twenty-five, but she monitors and shepherds her energy so that her working days begin at eight and end at eight. If she eats right and exercises, she says, the consciousness of the wisewoman is always with her.

EMPTYING AND REFILLING

Mastering the physical and psychological challenges of the Change might be seen as a test, a necessary exercise, forcing us to look ahead and accept the new perspective coming into view. Each major life passage entails emptying and refilling. It is particularly literal, and poignant, during menopause. There is first the gushing, like the reddening of a dying tree as it blazes out in its final autumn with a flaming canopy. As we move into post-menopause, we are emptied of the menses that has dominated our reproductive phase. We are reduced to basics, forced to lie fallow. Within that emptiness, watered by tears over the surrender of our magical powers of birthing, if we hold fast through the dark night of unknowing, we can discover our greater fertility. Contemplating the face of nature reminds us of our responsibility for creation and protection of the earth and of earth wisdom. While men are programmed by evolution to live short, high-performance lives, women are wired to endure.

The greatest boon of menopause is that it forces us to tune in to our body's needs and quirks and to stay intimately tuned. It is, after all, the house in which we will dwell for the rest of our days, and we will be comfortable in it only if we learn how to turn down the stress on our heart and keep the mineral turning over in our bone. A new balance must be struck between output and input. What is needed for replenishment? For some women it's the decision to take a four-day weekend every six weeks—to climb a mountain, look at the sea, or simply drop out with music or books—whatever it takes to empty one's cares and find the calm for centering. For others, the Change is the signal to change unhealthy eating habits, stop smoking, invest in serious exercise, and learn what their body needs to feel good. For those who are already exercise habitués, they may need to balance aerobic exercise, which is demanding of the body, with yoga or meditation.

But more than that, of all the passages, the Change of Life is a process of emptying and refilling that requires a new companionship between mind and body.

I believe it is vital to develop a future self in the mind's eye. She is our better nature, with bits and pieces of the most vital mature women we have known or read about and wish to emulate. If we are going to go gray, or white, we can pick out the most elegant white-haired woman we know and incorporate that element into our own inner picture. The more clearly we visualize our ideal future self, admire her indomitable skeleton and the groves of experience that make up the map of her face, the more comfortable we will be with moving into her container.

An inspiring public model of wisewoman power is Elizabeth Cady Stanton. As one who pursued justice for women well into her eighties, Stanton was living proof of her belief, which was eloquently recounted in her autobiography:

"The heyday of a woman's life is the shady side of fifty, when the vital forces heretofore expended in other ways are garnered in the brain, when their thoughts and sentiments flow out in broader channels, when philanthropy takes the place of family selfishness, and when from the depths of poverty and suffering the wail of humanity grows as pathetic to their ears as once was the cry of their own children."

Postscript

*T*o mark my own rite of passage through menopause, *I gave myself a few days alone in the mountains. I wanted to honor my graduation into the new stage of Second Adulthood and to reward my body for all the days it had already served me. On the last day I awoke after a full refreshment of sleep on a nearly empty stomach and opened the curtains to a dazzling sight.*

The moon hung full over the hills. Unhurried by the day's first light, she reveled in her fullness. I went outside to sit in contemplation of her, and we faced each other in utter equanimity: She who had pulled the tides of my inner sea for 450-some months, powerfully, capriciously, violently, now had relaxed her hold on me and left my waters calm as a lagoon after a tropical storm. Emptied, I sat there in the twig-brushing breeze and savored the quiet aliveness that had come to me at last.

The moon began to sink, and I rose to fill my container

with the new day. I felt pulled to hike up the face of a mountain considered sacred by shamans who once ministered to the Indians of this valley. Even then this mountain radiated a spiritual energy that drew those with the most subtle attunedness. Here the shamans marked rites of passage and performed rituals for birth and rites of fertility. It seemed an apt place to create my own ritual for marking this third blood mystery of a woman's life.

On the approach to the mountain my senses were quickened by each patch of herbs—the snap of sage, the tickle of thyme, the melancholy of rosemary, and what was that? The swoon of honeysuckle? Soon the scents were left behind as the bare rock and silver stubble of the foothills asserted their elemental simplicity. No frills here, only endurance. The wild herbs and grasses and desert flowers have the look of all healthily aging things: silvery gray, with strong roots, their flexible stems able to bend in the storm, their flowers calculated to bloom in the fissures between. All that is most creative and startling in life springs up in the cracks between.

As I followed the spiraling path up the mountain, lifting out of myself, I felt my inner world merging with the outer world. It was a world of silences, broken only by the munch of footfall on the crumbled earth and the sucking of Santa Ana winds. The moon was still in place. All at once the sun carved a dipper out of the opposite mountain and ladled its liquid gold down the face. The pure energy was almost overpowering. A sparkler of red and green spun for a few seconds in a mirrored circle beneath the great ball.

Then I sat for an undeciphered period of time in meditation on the brow of the far mountain. Honor the mellowed silence in you, *I thought.* Mark these moments

when you are aware of not doing, not wanting, not pre-
paring for the next activity, but simply filling with the
moment. *The more still I became, the more I was able to
feel the earth traveling beneath me. I could see the sun
hung over one horizon, ravishing, while behind me, in
exactly the same position over the shadow side of the mountain, the moon was fading. The cymbals of day and night
hung in perfect equipoise. The wind quieted.*

*Then all at once I felt a surge of energy. Warm, whirling,
giddy, it moved upward, setting words to buzzing in my
brain. A sense of such exultation filled me. It was as if the
hourglass had been turned over and the crystals of creative
energy were flowing in reverse—from womb to mind. I
couldn't wait to get back to my laptop, my writing . . . my
passion.*

*We are all pilgrims together, finding our way, but the
markers we lay along the trail will beckon future generations to even longer lives. Let us mark the way well. Filled
with new life and license, let us bring the cymbals of light
and shadow together and begin again.*

Index

ABOUT THE AUTHOR

GAIL SHEEHY is the author of nine books, including her landmark work, *Passages*. In a 1991 Library of Congress and Book-of-the-Month Club survey of the books that have most influenced people's lives, *Passages* was listed in the top ten. It was followed by *Pathfinders*, another bestseller by Ms. Sheehy, which, drawing on a study of sixty thousand Americans, presented portraits of men and women who emerged victorious from the predictable crises or accidents of life. Ms. Sheehy has also written *Lovesounds* (a novel), *Speed Is of the Essence, Panthermania, Hustling, Spirit of Survival, Character: America's Search for Leadership,* and *The Man Who Changed the World: The Lives of Mikhail S. Gorbachev.*

Ms. Sheehy was one of the original contributors to *New York* magazine and is now a contributing editor of *Vanity Fair*. She is the mother of two daughters and lives in New York City with her husband, publisher and editor Clay Felker.